THE Sexercise BOOK

THE Sexercise BOOK

FIT MAGAZINE PRESENTS

by Kym Herrin with Richard Benyo

Herrin, Kym.
    The sexercise book.

    1. Sex instruction for women. 2. Exercise—Physiological
aspects.   I. Benyo, Richard.   II. Title.
HQ46.H47   1982   613.9'6   82-13786
ISBN 0-89037-226-8

Photography by David Keith

Contents

Contents

Introduction

Sexercise is an exercise program specifically designed to heighten sexual fulfillment.

It is based on the knowledge that no one is perfect. And it recognizes that no one can attain perfection, but that most people make genuine attempts in that direction.

Examine yourself sexually. Be honest with yourself. Do you feel that you are in shape physically to fully enjoy sex? Do you feel you could use more sexual energy? How smoothly and how well does your body move? Did your curiosity at the possibility of finding a road to better sex inspire you to pick up this book? Or did you just want to look at the pictures? Seriously, though, does your body exhibit the flexibility that it used to? Do you often find your body fagging out during sex before your desire is sated?

The fact that you picked up this book indicates an interest in working toward your sexual potential. And that desire to improve is the motive force that makes Sexercise work. It is fortunate that one's sexual adventures serve to further fan the flames of desire, literally making that desire an inexhaustible source of sexual energy. This is the bedrock of Sexercise.

Whether your lovemaking is frenetic or languid, your body is called upon to perform in positions and at angles that it does not practice every day. This, in turn, places certain limitations on the enjoyment and fulfillment you derive from the experience. In other words, if you do not practice sit-ups in your daily life, the basic missionary position, if you are female, is going to be quite exhausting — and often that exhaustion comes just before you and your partner reach the precipice of orgasm. The purpose of Sexercise, then, is to enable that needed flexibility and strength to help you make the great leap.

Sexercise is not, however, a book on sexual therapy. It assumes that you are normally active sexually, and does not purport to have answers to why someone fails to engage in sex on a regular basis. It does not examine sexual deviations and does not shed light on sexual dysfunction. It is not a manual for couples having difficulties in their relationships. And it is certainly not meant to be a medical treatise on sexuality and copulation.

Rather, it *is* a guide to getting to know your body in a sexual sense. It is also a guide to getting to know the body of your male sex partner. It is a program of developing strength, endurance and flexibility so that you can function more comfortably within a sexual situation — and so that your body can take you where you have never gone before in sexual experiences.

I think you would agree that if you are physically fit and toned, sex can be enhanced. I enjoy watching a well-toned and fit man who moves purposefully, exhibiting a certain air of confidence in his body movements. I don't mean he must be a man who threatens to burst his shirt every time he raises his arm to hail a taxi. I'll admit that I have a preference for men who are well-built, athletic, and who have a physique that leans more toward a fullback than a marathoner. But I can appreciate — and feel a certain warmth building within me for — a man who is toned and moves well, whether I will ever personally know him or not. It is the same appreciation that comes from watching the restless prancing of that beautiful steed in *"The Black Stallion."*

For too long, too many people have felt that it was either too late in life or too much work to become more flexible, to enhance body strength and to build endurance. The fitness movement, fortunately, has changed the minds of millions of people in that regard. People who once were not athletically inclined are now running marathons, playing racquetball, taking aerobic dance and Jazzercise classes — and loving it. That psychological barrier that had kept many people from leading physically active lives has been breached, and it now seems as though it was merely a mental stumbling block.

I have examined my own life with a view toward physical fitness and have read a small mountain of books on yoga, isotonics, weightlifting for men and women, postnatal exercises from women, stretching techniques, etc. From my experiences with all of these disciplines, I have fashioned specific exercises that focus on developing, strengthening and loosening muscles that relate to sex. When you combine all these disciplines, you literally touch upon every system in the body that relates in any way to sexual fulfillment.

You will find that your body can adapt to this program with relative ease. In contrast to exercise programs that progress hastily or are too difficult, you may go at your own pace, and the exercises are easy to master.

Introduction

Once you have integrated the Sexercise program into your daily life, your day will seem empty without it. As you begin to see — and feel — the results, and realize the potential for continuing to create a more invigorated, sensuous you, the exercises will take on greater significance.

I do want to stress that this book will feature straight-talk about sex, sexual positions and sexual adventures that you can incorporate into your life. The main emphasis of Sexercise is to increase your potential to express love, physically. It is to make sex more comfortable and more enjoyable — and to make it more creative.

This book is written with the knowledge that sex is something that can be improved upon throughout your life. No one is born with sexual techniques or sexual capacities that are terrific. You learn to be sexually sensitive and adept, and to bring the most possible pleasure to yourself and your man.

Sexercise can improve even the best lovers. And remember, the way the best lovers became so good was by maintaining the ability to continue learning. Sexercise and making love are based upon strength, flexibility, endurance, tone — and patience.

• *Strength* — in the limbs, stomach, pelvic region, buttocks, back, feet, hands and neck, so that your sexual moves are controlled, natural and comfortable to yourself and your lover. Strength, so that there is nothing tentative about your role in sex.

• *Flexibility* — so that you can instigate as well as react to any direction your sex play takes. This includes comfortably getting into, and staying in, positions that are exquisitely pleasurable, until you are ready to move to another equally creative position. Flexibility, so that there is no position or angle that intimidates you. This opens up whole new worlds of adventure and pleasure.

• *Endurance* — so that your body will not give out before your enthusiasm does. Endurance, so that you can follow one sexual adventure with another and another. Endurance, so that you can stretch and hold your sexual adventures at the limits of endurance and, once completed, come back for more.

• *Tone* — so that your body can be at its highest efficiency and best appearance, giving visual and tactile pleasure to your lover, and satisfaction to you every time you pass a mirror. Each of us has another, and better

self inside the person we are. By taking advantage of Sexercise to tone yourself, you can reach your full potential, and when you do, there is a certain glow of self-confidence and well-being that radiates from within. That glow and assurance can be a real turn-on, as far as sex goes. No matter how near you are to your potential, there is always that little bit more that you can urge from yourself, and that can make a world of difference to you — and to your lover.

• *Patience* — so that you can begin a Sexercise program *today*, and maintain it throughout the rest of your life. Patience to realize that change, even when you work at it diligently, does not come overnight; but that, when worked at regularly, patience most certainly does come.

This book is built on the integration of all these elements. When they all come into play simultaneously, Sexercise moves beyond the capacity for better sex. It causes your entire life to be infused with a new glow, a new level of self-esteem, a new confidence in your power and potential as a human being working at the maximum level.

The first chapter of this book is a fairly quick, and certainly simplified, examination of how your body functions. I have made it as *un*medical and as unstuffy as possible. I have also tried to make it as interesting as possible.

The body is a wonderful machine that we often take for granted. I don't mean that we forget its presence or that we totally ignore it. I mean that we seldom take a moment to contemplate the wonderful complexities of ourselves. We seldom stop and think how the simplest movement of the body is an incredible meshing of intricate and complex and mysterious interconnections between various body systems. The body is more marvelous than the galaxies that astound us when we peer into a telescope. But there I go, making it sound more complicated and complex than it need be. It is just that I get a little carried away by the captivating aspects of the human body. Your appreciation of some of its fantastic systems will make your lovemaking a more sensitive and knowledgeable act.

I've also included a chapter on Sexersaage, in which I've concentrated on creating a warm and sensitive session between lovers; it will become an unforgettable occasion, no matter what your previous experience — or lack of experience — with massage.

Another chapter is about Sexercise with your lover. It could also be referred to as Couples Sexercise. In this chapter, you can learn to develop certain muscle groups and body systems that are difficult to improve upon without a partner. In the process, the Sexercise can be a real turn-on.

Yet another chapter deals with unique exercises for the woman, which will develop the muscles surrounding her internal, sex-related organs. Often overlooked, the development of these muscles can have far-reaching benefits, from making specific sexual positions more comfortable, to gaining better muscle control in the vagina, to learning to ease menstrual cramps. These are very important muscles to the completely sexual woman, and it is incredible how few women take the time to develop them — or even know that they can be exercised like any other muscles in the body.

Sexercises in sequences that can be done to music are covered in one chapter. I've included sequences with various tempos and beats that work well with a variety of popular songs, which are available at your local record and tape store. Doing your Sexercise routine to music can convert it from exercise to a more enjoyable form of dance.

The backbone of the book, however, is chapters two, three and four.

In those chapters, Sexercise is divided into three categories, based on degree of difficulty:

1. *Casual Level.* Primarily a warmup and cooldown for experienced exercisers, and for novice exercisers who are interested in the proper development of strength and flexibility.

2. *Intimate Level.* More difficult than the Casual Level, with the assumption that you are coming to Sexercise with some strength and flexibility already built up from an ongoing physical fitness program. Also, the middle level toward which beginners can work.

3. *Intense Level.* Fairly difficult but satisfying Sexercise for the experienced exerciser, and for the Sexercise exerciser who has worked her way up through the two previous levels and who is aiming toward the ultimate.

While reading and using this book, always keep in mind that sex and Sexercise can best be appreciated and made to work for you if you approach it in a playful, positive way. Remember: exercise creates and restores energy; energy promotes the capacity for fitness; and fitness can be used effectively to heighten and generally enhance sexual performance.

Kym Herrin
Santa Barbara, California
September, 1982

CHAPTER 1

The Soft Machine

Science is enjoying a resurgence today. There are television specials on the complexities of the human heart, on satellite communications, on the workings of electricity and on how meteorology is still a guessing game. There are glossy magazines about science and technology, which tell us how astronomers discover distant planets they can't see even with the aid of a telescope, explain the computer's omnipresence and how it will guide our future, how animals — and ultimately people — can be cloned.

The first surge in scientific achievement in America came after the Russians beat us into space with the Sputnik satellite, at the end of the 1950s. America's educators then stressed learning the sciences, hoping that we could regain the lead in space and technology. During the 1960s our attention turned to internal unrest and the unpopular war in Southeast Asia; these events seemed to drain us of our interest in anything else. The 1970s saw us draw inward, paying a great deal of attention to ourselves; we took up fitness with a vengeance as we tried, by exercise, to ward off aging.

In the 1980s, there is evidence that beneficial health effects are being carried over from the exercise craze. We've seen heart disease, by far our number one cause of death in America, begin a decline for two reasons: the modern methods of treating — and saving — a heart attack victim, and because exercise has strengthened our hearts. Strong hearts are less susceptible to heart disease.

With the corresponding growth of science, we are seemingly on the verge of a Golden Age — a time of understanding ourselves, and of living longer and more satisfying lives. Recent medical advances as a result of scientific research are astounding. Doctors are performing heart-and-lung transplants in a single operation, a doctor in Pittsburgh is doing liver transplants, one of the most complex and difficult of all human organs to repair; and there is optimism that researchers are on the threshold of finding cures for certain types of cancer.

Our bodies, which we sometimes take for granted, and other times become obsessed with, continue to be sources of wonder for scientists. The more we learn about the body, the more fascinating it becomes to us. In simple terms, it is an organic machine. To the philosopher or the scientist, it is the most complex and wonderful machine known to man. To most of us, however, it is a machine not too unlike an automobile.

Most of us walk out to the garage or to the curb, open the door of our car, slide in, insert the key, turn it, wait a moment for the motor to turn, put the car into gear and take off. We do the simple maintenance checks. We occasionally check the oil and the coolant, add a little air to a tire if it looks low, and fill it with gasoline when it needs it. Some people *totally* simplify car maintenance by only concerning themselves with putting gasoline in the car when it's needed. The rest, they assume, will be taken care of when the car goes in for its twice-annual tune-up.

Someone who does not take care of his car is annoyed and surprised when it breaks down and leaves him stranded along a deserted country road late at night during a snowstorm. It is the "dumb car's fault" that it has bald rear tires, no anti-freeze/coolant in the engine, no windshield washer, a dry battery, it needs three quarts of oil in the crankcase, and the gasoline gauge reads "E."

A tow truck is called and the car is towed to a mechanic, who puts it back together as best he can, within the limits of the driver's checkbook and within the limits of what's left on the car that can be saved.

The human body, we've learned, is very similar. We let certain body systems go bad, we don't maintain the body with regular checkups, we let parts of it "rust" from disuse, and suddenly, one day, there is an ambulance outside and we're being taken to the hospital, where the doctors pore over us, digging around to see what can be saved.

The analogy between the human body and the automobile has its limitations, certainly. If you use the car frequently, parts begin to wear out. Marvelously, many human parts actually gain strength, function, flexibility and endurance if they are used frequently. In the human machine, that marvelous characteristic extends all the way to the brain, an item that doesn't even come as an option on the automble.

This discussion is, essentially, a lead-in to several important points:

1. The human body is very much finite, and certainly destructible, but few of us use it to its fullest or push it to reach its maximum potential.

2. There are certain things we can do that

can greatly improve our bodies; there are scientifically verifiable principles that can increase the strength, coordination, flexibility, tone and endurance of the human body.

3. A body coaxed to improve itself can enjoy far-reaching health/wellness benefits.

4. A healthy, toned, well-tuned body is capable of more fully enjoying all things in life, including sex; it can respond better, longer and more frequently, and its maximum development can serve to stimulate your sex partner. Sex is a prime motivating force in the life of a human being, and sex increases in enjoyment and in fulfillment the more comfortable you are engaging in it; a supple, well-toned body can react and interact more comfortably than one that is inflexible, staid, flaccid, moribund, tired, inept, and running on only half its cylinders.

5. A simple appreciation of your body will not necessarily lead to narcissism, although it may lead to a more intimate friendship and alliance between who you are as a person and what your body contributes to you as a person.

6. Occasional contemplations of your body's marvelous workings and how, when you treat it well, it responds in kind, can lead to philosophical insights and a greater appreciation for life.

* * *

The title of this chapter is "The Soft Machine," which differentiates the extraordinary human body and mind from man-made machines. Machines are molded from metals and plastics; they are "Hard Machines," made to withstand the rigors of Earth's environment.

Perhaps because the human body has a functional life extending far beyond the seemingly indestructible Hard Machines, we should learn something on a philosophical level about some errors in our thinking. Of course, it's a little late to radically change the fundamentals of producing a machine. We can't suddenly convert to soft materials. Besides, it would be nearly impossible now to learn to be comfortable with an electric toaster that felt and looked like a human breast, or a typewriter that in every way except function resembled a female buttocks. Sounds like a scene from Woody Allen's *"Everything You Wanted To Know About Sex, Part II."*

"The Soft Machine" refers to our organic structure. The bones that make up our skeleton, certainly, are not exactly soft; however, in the early years of life our bones are more pliable and flexible than they are in old age, when they become downright brittle. But everything else in us — compared to such machines as cars, elevators, microwave ovens, massive earthmovers, electric toothbrushes, etc. — is fairly soft. That quality of being soft and pliant also allows us to grow and move and go through various changes.

A 1982 Z-28 Camaro will look much the same ten years from now as it does today in

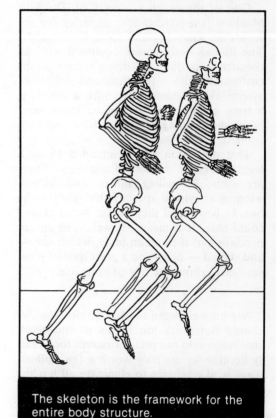

The skeleton is the framework for the entire body structure.

the dealer's showroom; sure, it will show some signs of wear and tear. But it will have essentially the same dimensions, the same weight, the same shape and, if the engine is fine-tuned and well-maintained, it should run pretty much as it did when you drove it away from the dealer's.

The 1982 model of yourself, however, will undergo many changes over the next ten years. That's an inherent trap of and tribute to a soft machine. Sit on a sofa doing nothing but eating bonbons and watching soap operas, and you'll at first see some subtle changes that, as they gain momentum, become quite pronounced. Dimensions, weight and shape change. Nothing works as it did a decade before. But that's a result of the do-nothing trap.

The tribute to The Soft Machine, the flip side of the coin so to speak, is that the body can be molded and improved. It can be made tougher, sleeker, more flexible, able to astound its owner. Feed it properly, exercise it, give it a chance to enjoy life and its place in life, and it will flourish. This certainly includes flourishing sexually.

One of the enticing aspects of The Soft Machine is its tremendous capacity for enjoying its sensuality and using its sexuality. The human body comes equipped with all the dealer options. It doesn't have to be customized with a few thousand dollars of aftermarket equipment, as with a car. It is merely a matter of getting to know your body, maintaining it, developing it and then using it.

This discussion is not intended to be a lengthy treatise on human anatomy. There are some bestselling books and award-winning television specials that glorify the human body, and they do far better than I could here. It is meant, however, as an appreciation of the human body, which can — and should — bring you a great deal of pleasure throughout the rest of your life.

*   *   *

We have all heard the admonition that we should not think too highly of ourselves, that we should not prize ourselves too greatly because we are only worth a few dollars. That is, if one were to eliminate all but the minerals and other substances that comprise our bodies, there would be little left of value. Ten years ago, that value came to a bit more than two dollars per body; with inflation, the price tag on each of us has increased modestly, while the contents are no different.

Every time I hear how little we are worth in the raw materials market, it gives me a greater appreciation of each person's value. For two dollars, or even ten-dollars-worth of materials, The Soft Machine that you get is a pretty incredible bargain. Manufacturers can't build a good toaster for under ten bucks, much less a human. But for that price we get a thinking, speaking, breathing, moving machine that has a warranty good for sixty or seventy years. Pretty incredible.

To consider the human body in all its glory and complexity, let's once again use the analogy of the automobile. Let's also again use the 1982 Z-28 Camaro, a sleek-looking machine.

The car is constructed mainly from raw materials: rubber, glass, metal. There are also man-made materials: plastics, synthetic rubber, fabric. And there are fluids: brake fluid, gasoline, crankcase oil, battery acid, axle grease.

The car functions by the careful integration of various systems. There is an electrical system, with the battery as the base of operations; turn the key and a relay is activiated, which allows the flow of electricity from the battery to the starter motor and from the battery to the coil; as the starter motor turns, it moves the engine parts. As they move, the charge going through the coil (which intensifies the electrical charge), and from there to the spark plugs, will be enough to ignite the gasoline forced into the cylinder heads by the carburetor. The motor will then start. When the battery was engaged, its stored electricity was also tapped to feed the radio and the cigarette lighter and the other electrically operated apparatuses in the car. All this would soon drain the battery's reserve of electrical power, so to feed electricity back into the battery and to keep it charged, the motor's running also drives a fan belt, which then turns either an alternator or a generator. The car also has many basic mechanical systems, such as the transmission (which changes power from one direction to another to turn the wheels), pressure plate, parking brake, etc.

The human body is constructed of various raw materials: calcium, potassium, magnesium, iron, water, acids. There are no synthetic materials, unless you've had dental work or corrective surgery.

The human body also functions by the careful integration of various systems. Hold your hand in front of your face and clench it into a fist. Not to overly complicate the movement, but the action of closing your fist was the culmination of a series of events happening very, very rapidly. The signal to close it came from the brain. The brain is the control center of the body. Whatever your body does (save involuntary muscle contractions), it does through commands issued by the brain. Even withdrawing your hand from contact with a hot stove involves a signal being sent from your hand to your brain. The nerve endings in the hand have picked up a very uncomfortable signal of TOO MUCH HEAT and your brain sends back a command of: "Well, stupid, take it off — as fast as you can!"

Signals travel from your hand to your brain (and from your brain back to your hand) through a series of nerves that function on a chemical and electrical system. The signal to clench your fist travels from the brain, down through the spinal cord, branches out along your arm, and reaches your hand. The signal causes the muscles on the inside of the fingers to contract and bring them together into a fist. The muscles are attached to the bones of the fingers. There are ligaments between the bones. They allow bones to move and hold them together. If there were no ligaments, all of our bones would fall to the floor and we'd look more like a six-inch-high glob of Jello.

When we are done making a fist, we can again open the hand by sending signals to the abductor muscles to contract, thus pulling the hand open. Muscles do their work by contracting. But each muscle that contracts must have a companion muscle that works in the opposite direction, so that once the first muscle contracts it doesn't get stuck there. Hold your hand in front of your face with the edge of your thumb in front of your nose. Now, slowly move your hand and arm to the left, noting the muscles in your arm that are working; next, move it slowly to the right; feel the alternate muscles in your arm coming into play? If you are very attentive, you can feel the instant when the muscles change function.

Let's jump back to the example of your hand coming in contact with a hot stove. The sensation is a painful one. It is painful because the nerve endings in your hand are telling your brain that it is painful. (This brings up a point about dinosaurs. They had such rudimentary brains — actually ganglia — and signals had to travel so far, that if man had been alive in that era, he could have sneaked up from behind, cut off the dinosaur's tail, and the creature would have bled to death by the time the signal got to its brain that it had lost its tail.) If you were to have an accident in which the nerves coming from your hand to your brain were cut, your brain wouldn't get the signal that your hand

was being burned on the stove, you'd feel no pain and within a few minutes you'd have a fried hand. This is one of the principles used in anesthesia. When you go into a dentist's office to have a tooth extracted, and you receive a local anesthetic like novocaine, the drug blocks the nerves from that portion of your mouth that would normally be sending cries of distress to your brain to register pain. Intoxication has much the same effect; as a drug, alcohol numbs the brain, so the signals announcing that you dropped a wine bottle on your foot will take longer to get to

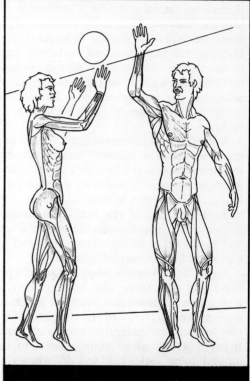

The muscles account for the body's mobility and strength.

the brain.

The nerve endings in the hands (and in every other portion of the body; your skin, after all, is a huge sensation receptor) are not placed there just so you can protect your hands from becoming injured or fried. They are also there to send pleasurable sensations to the brain.

When you stroke the inside of the thighs of your lover, you can cause the movement to be excruciatingly sensuous for him. The signals transmitted from the touch of your hands against your lover's skin move up through your fingers, your arm, your spinal cord, and from there to your brain. In the brain, they spark ideas, memories and impressions of your lover. The sense of touch is amplified and made more exciting because you are touching the skin of someone you love.

But we are jumping slightly ahead of ourselves. This explanation of how sensations travel along nerve endings to reach the brain, where they knock for admission and demand a reaction once they're inside, is not meant to bog down our discussion of Sexercise. However, it is the basis of the entire book, because you must understand something of how the body works in order to improve its function. When we discuss Sexersaage, for example, the importance of sensations and nerve endings will become doubly important. And as we discuss the three levels of Sexercise, the importance of coordination between muscle groups will become profound.

As we've already mentioned, there are many well-written anatomy books, ranging in difficulty from the layman's guide to the medical researcher's textbook. It is fascinating to follow the workings of the human body. I urge each of you to take an interest in your body, from the standpoint of making and keeping it at its functional best, and to understand its wonderful complexity.

Again, as we've mentioned and as we'll remind you repeatedly: one of your body's wonders, as opposed to a machine, is that in most instances, the more you use parts of it, the greater its potential endurance and strength. Don't allow your muscles to lie around doing nothing. If you do, when you make demands of them they will respond slowly and become sore quickly — and that includes the times you make love.

We will emphasize repeated physical activity to strengthen, flex, tone and build endurance in muscle groups. By making physical demands of your body, you come to know it better and appreciate it more. Also, your senses become more keen through use and more atuned to the signals they are receiving from outside sources — especially from your lover.

While making love, have you ever noticed a particular touch or sensation hit you in a uniquely stimulating way, and later, when you lay back and tried to re-create it, you couldn't? Sometimes you can't simulate a sensation because you are so involved in lovemaking that your sensations are seemingly in neutral. They're ready to follow whatever course the lovemaking takes. But with practice and training, you can become more intimate with your body. And by doing that, you'll be able to read and store for later use sensation signals as they happen. You'll be able to re-create the same exciting or satisfying sensation you experienced and had forgotten before you were practicing Sexercise.

Like learning to walk or talk or write, lovemaking is an activity where repetition is the mother of expertise. However, taking an almost academic approach to lovemaking, and consciously training yourself physically for enjoying it more fully, does not detract from its romance.

It is, in fact, the incredible capacity of the human mind to accumulate knowledge and to store it for future use that potentially enhances everything we do. Consider sex. Whereas an animal's sex life is almost universally linked to breeding, the human being takes a far more complex and varied approach. And it is an approach that is continually being enhanced by pleasurable memories of previous sexual encounters. Memorable sexual movements, positions and sequences of embraces and caresses, when re-created, can intensify the pleasure of a sexual experience.

*   *   *

I am constantly astonished at the capacity of the human body to adapt to what we require of it. This adaptation is improved if we take time to learn about and understand our body, and to become intimately familiar with its unique qualities.

Some people can adapt much faster than others to a particular physical activity. I'm sure you can remember — I know I do — that there were some kids in the high-school physical education class who were Boy Wonders at every sport that came along. Sometimes they were better than you, even though it was their first encounter with a sport. They were the same types as the outstanding performers you met in music class, shop, home economics and algebra. And in the back seat of a Chevy on Friday nights. Occasionally, there was a person so "cool" that he was outstanding in virtually everything he tried; he was the envy of everyone in school. But let's be honest, those of us who had no talent hated him for that reason.

But the point is this: virtually everyone, by repetition, study, and practice, became sufficiently adept at the activity to pass and move on to bigger and better things. I know several people from high school who were late bloomers. Now they're excellent tennis players or runners or pianists. They could probably perform rings around the intuitively talented person — simply because they stayed with it. They genuinely enjoyed what they were learning, they were patient with themselves and their activity became an integral part of their lives.

The same goes for exercise and sex.

The Z-28 car we keep using as an example has certain limitations that are, because of technology and production costs, programed into it. Rev the engine too high (even after it has been broken in) and you'll have pistons exploding through the hood and the bottom end of the engine scattered on the asphalt. No matter what you do to the car, short of adding a great amount of aftermarket high-performance parts, which make the car something other than a Z-28, its capabilities are limited.

With the human body, The Soft Machine, this is not so. The body's pliability, softness and flexibility is one of its greatest strengths! No matter what your condition at this very moment, from accomplished sedentary slob to triathlete, the body is capable of improving — given proper treatment and training.

The same is true of sex. No one is born a great lover. It is something that is learned by intuition, by practice or by both. No matter what sexual level you are currently at, you can still improve. You can do that by improving your physical condition. It has a profound effect upon all aspects of your sex life, from technique to attractiveness.

Let's talk first about developing physically. Then, in the next segment, we'll talk about how that can be effectively translated to sex. A surprising number of people who *do* exercise regularly manage to forget the simple principles that underline that entire lifestyle. If you are just getting into exercising, you can easily overlook, forget or ignore some of the basic principles. We'll lay down the basic laws here:

1. The body is a highly adaptable machine. Give it an unfamiliar task and it will make valiant attempts to accommodate you.

Give it the same tasks the next day and it will not do as well. It may, in fact, break down. Why? Because adaptability is not a one-way street. For each task you subject your body to, you must also give your body ample rest, a time to recover before repeating the same task at a slightly more demanding level.

2. Exercise is an adaptive activity. You begin exercise at a set level, pushing your body slightly beyond its former capacity, and then back off. Allow the body to recover before stressing it again.

3. In order to adapt, a body must be given tasks regularly, with programed rest periods between; exercise is a task very agreeable to the human body.

4. If regularity is interrupted for any reason, the body must be allowed to backtrack to a comfortable level, because to pick up where it left off invites injury.

5. The most common mistake in exercising, made by the novice and veteran, is *over*training, not *under*training.

So what does this list infer?

It infers that *anyone* can exercise, because as the body is supremely adaptable, so exercising is adaptable to any body. It also infers that exercising is both hard and easy.

The hardest part of exercising is not the exercise itself but taking the first step, making the commitment to do it. It's hard to look in the mirror and say, ''Yeah, today is the day I'm going to start exercising, and I'm going to do it wisely and stick with it.''

The other difficulty is to be regular, to exercise on those days when you don't feel motivated, because those are the days when it can be the most valuable, both physically and mentally. The easy part of exercising is doing the exercises.

All those books and PE instructors who told you exercise is difficult were way off base. They made the mistake of trying to address groups of people instead of individuals, and exercise — like sex — is very much an individual activity. Think back to PE classes. A class was organized in line after line of pimple-faced and awkward kids. The instructor stood at the front of the class and led the entire group through calisthenics. Calisthenics form the backbone of all exercising, and they can be fun, but they weren't then. The instructor turned us off to calisthenics by forcing us into one mold, as though each of us were at the same ability level. They told us to do a certain number of repetitions for a certain duration and we had no choice in the matter. No wonder our bodies protested and tried to talk us out of liking exercises.

A class of forty high school kids covers a lot of territory in terms of muscular development and physical maturity. The problem was not just with the ones who were overweight. An average kid might be able to do eighteen jumping jacks comfortably, but the instructor took you through thirty jumping jacks. The twelve extra jumping jacks were a negative experience. Add to that the five extra push-ups, the five sit-ups, plus the two additional laps around the perimeter of the gym, and the seeds for a serious attitude problem against exercise have been planted. By the time you left high school, after all those gym classes, exercise was a real turn-off.

That's why it is important to:

1. Give exercising a chance.

2. Exercise at a level and frequency comfortable to *your* body.

3. Establish a regular schedule and stick with it.

4. Be patient with your body. Don't expect results overnight.

5. Do not become impatient and push yourself too far, too fast.

6. Don't think you must join an exercise class, if you prefer working out alone.

7. If you join an exercise class, be honest with yourself about your current fitness level and do not join a class too advanced for you. If the class is too easy, you can always make it work for you by adding a few more of each of the exercises after everyone else is through.

8. If your exercising is interrupted, do not throw up your hands in despair and quit; instead, back up a few steps. Depending on how long you are away from exercise, repeat some of the levels you've already covered. Allow your body time to re-adapt itself. Go forward from there.

9. Learn to listen to your body. Your exercise schedule need not be followed to the letter. If you have had a particularly hard, long or stressful day, be prepared to modify your workout. Make it easier than you had planned. It should refresh you instead of stress you. Once you exhaust yourself, it can take up to a week of rest to get back to a level where exercising is fun. So, don't exhaust yourself and risk staleness.

10. Learn the importance of rest. As we've already discussed, the human body develops and improves by a process of adaptation. Exercise exerts physical stress upon the body; the body responds by handling it. This response has pushed the body to a slightly higher capacity to accept stress, but in order to rebuild from the stress before it can be pushed to the next plateau, the body needs rest. This is why, at the start, you will want to exercise only every other day. Once you are farther along, or if you are already physically fit, you can exercise almost every day. But be sure you vary the exercises and that you do not stress the same muscles several days in a row. This is what runners refer to as The Hard/Easy Method. Work hard one day to stress the body, and do an easy workout (or none at all) the next day to recover. If you were to graph your exercise stress level daily, the line might look like a flight of stairs. Occasionally, you might want to set aside an entire week for easy exercise.

* * *

So how does all of this apply to sex? There are many parallels between exercise and sex. Recall the high school gym classes, and where I jokingly mentioned that some students were very adept at learning things in the back seats of Chevvies. Let's face it, back in high school a few people were naturally good in sports and a few got to first base with the opposite sex just as easily. Some of my friends never spent a weekend night with their feet on the ground.

But just because someone got an early start doesn't mean that he ever improved beyond that point. Most people who get started with sex later in life are equally adept, and can quickly develop some terrific techniques.

We assume that you have a sex life — a normal one at that — and that you want to improve it physically. By improving physically, we mean being more flexible (to assume more interesting and enjoyable positions), stronger and with greater endurance (to get maximum pleasure).

Sex should be fun. To be fun it must be comfortable for both partners. Fitness benefits comfort. Fitness can reduce the strain of taking certain sexual positions. For example, women commonly find it uncomfortable having their legs spread wide for a long time. Obviously, women only find themselves exercising in this manner during lovemaking. The same applies to men. A man assumes sexual positions that he does not assume at any other time in day-to-day living. So he may tire quickly in such positions.

Sexercise does more than give you the ability to better hold a sex position. It also causes other subtle changes.

A fitness program can alter the way that you perceive your body. There are some people who are fanatics about their bodies, about how they look. Some of them take it to extremes. They spend all their time powdering themselves and applying cosmetics to *hide* their flaws. Both men and women are affected this way. Rather than covering up, they should be exercising, working to bring out their best physical attributes. Once you begin to get fit, you positively glow. You exude good health. Your eyes sparkle, there is a freshness to your face, to the way you walk, to your skin. Make-up pales by comparison. And there is a vibrant sex appeal to the fit person. I've seen some mind-boggling "before" and "after" photos of middle-aged men and women who had gone from sedentary to physically fit. They were able to recapture the body tone and fitness of their youth. Even though these "new" people were fully clothed, you could still see the improvements by looking at the photos.

This physical metamorphosis is especially true of women I've known. They suddenly decide they want a change, and now they're running, taking yoga classes and doing regular exercises.

Nor is the change purely physical. If you are in good condition, if your muscles are toned, and if you are fit, you gain self-confidence and a sense of self-esteem creeps into your mannerisms, your speech, the way you walk and the way you hold your body. I know many men and women in their thirties who say that they are in better shape today than they were ten years ago in college. That is a bonus of living in the 1980s. Men and women reaching thirty needn't feel they face only encroaching physical deterioration. Rather than sitting around waiting to die, you can get up, move around and start a regular program to fight physical deterioration. And it's socially acceptable to play and work up a sweat in your middle-age years.

This is not to say that the physically fit are better lovers. There are some pretty unfit people with some very good sexual techniques. But the fit have the *potential* to be so much better sexually than the unfit — there's almost no comparison.

CHAPTER 2
Casual Sexercises

If I had a minute in Hawaii for every time I've heard, "I tried to follow an exercise plan, but I just can't seem to get it all together," I could live on Maui year-round. Amazingly, that's the reason I hear most when I ask someone why he or she doesn't exercise. After gathering the details, the catch-all reason of "I can't do them" breaks down into some definite patterns:

1. I've tried exercises, and although I can fake it through the really basic stuff, I'm overwhelmed by some of the more difficult ones.

2. I can't seem to motivate myself to do exercises regularly.

3. I don't like to sweat — it's unladylike.

4. I still have a hang-up against exercising from having to do those dumb calisthenics in high school.

It is not difficult to understand their reasons, but they just aren't good enough to prevent you from engaging in a regular exercise program — especially when in so doing, you can noticeably improve your sex life.

Let's deal with number three first. Women are human beings, just like men. Women can and do sweat. Some are reluctant to do it in public, and some even express revulsion for sweating in private, as though it were dirty or demeaning.

The contention that ladies do not sweat seems to have come from a class of people who sought any means they could to separate themselves from the toilers of the world. They felt that to sweat was lowly and common, and that to be a lady was to be everything that a common toiler or worker was not. Imagine the willpower it takes to maintain your status as a lady in the middle of summer in New Orleans when even the trees around you are dripping from the humidity that hangs in the air. You feel like you're being smothered in a warm, wet blanket. Many of those social barriers, which included sweating, have long since broken down, and some of the "best" families are now finding it agreeable to engage in exercise for the sake of the "old bod."

Actually, sweating is essential for maintaining a constant body temperature. Sweating occurs when the body attempts to cool itself. Often the body's temperature goes up because the outside temperature is high, but it's usually because the body is working or exercising. The body's inner temperature will climb to a point where it must react (sweat) or face serious problems. If the body cannot cool itself, its core temperature rises and can cause serious internal damage.

Some women, besides being psychologically reluctant to sweat, have difficulty getting their bodies to trigger the sweating mechanism. Sweating resembles exercising: it is partly a learned technique. While the body is quite capable of sweating, just as it is quite capable of doing basic exercises without any previous training, there is a process of adaptation. The body must learn to sweat on cue, to anticipate when the cooling mechanism is going to be needed. If you watch marathon runners training, you'll see that they "break a sweat" relatively early in a run. This is learned by the body. After training for many months, their bodies have learned that when running begins it will probably go on for a while. The body, that wonderfully adaptive organism, anticipates that long period of running. The body accounts for the cooling that will be required of it and, as a result, triggers the sweating/cooling mechanism very early in the exercise. Thus the marathoner's body more effectively maintains a stable temperature during the workout. The untrained person who goes for a run will likely begin perspiring later than the trained runner. He would probably continue sweating long after the marathoner had stopped sweating. That's because his unfit body is playing catch-up, trying desperately to get the cooling mechanism going, and then, because it is less efficient, keeping it going to eliminate all that built-up heat. Once a person begins exercising regularly, the process of sweating will naturally become more atuned to the activity, and sweating will begin to occur as an adjunct to the exercising.

If you still have a hang-up about sweating, you'll be glad to know that, besides being a cooling mechanism, it also helps cleanse the body of dirt and bacteria. There isn't a soap or cleansing agent that can get down into the pores and clean them out as well as a good sweat. Bacteria and dirt are eliminated through the millions of microscopic pores in your skin. A shower after a workout, then, is a very good way of cleansing the skin, especially if you begin the shower with warm water, soap down, and then gradually reduce the water temperature. The cooler water closes the pores; this helps prevent small particles of dirt from entering the opened pores after the shower and soap-down.

Now let's tackle the bad memories of high-school calisthenics. I'll have to be honest, and admit that for some of you, the gym classes were probably such a total turn-off that overcoming your dread of exercise will be a real uphill battle. To go at ridding yourself of all those bad memories you might try a simple exercise program, going at your own speed, starting at a level that you can easily handle, and doing it in the most pleasant environment you can imagine. There is nothing wrong, by the way, with starting your new exercise program in the privacy of your home, when there is no one else around; you don't even have to tell anyone you're doing it until you're good and ready. I've found that some of the most refreshing times of my life have been after a particularly good workout that I did completely alone, and at a speed that fit my mood that day. By the time I walked into the shower, I felt a real glow about the day, and after those exercise sessions a shower feels as sensuous as the gentle stroke of your lover.

But I'm getting carried away. My point is that no matter how negative your previous exercising experiences, it is a completely different world when you are in charge of the session. Give it a try, and please don't look at it in terms of gym, calisthenics, something you *have* to do, or group participation. Do it for yourself. You deserve to give yourself a second chance at exercising.

Purging the old stigma of gym class and developing a new image of exercising has a lot to do with motivation. But motivation is a very important part of exercising, even to someone who has very positive feelings about it.

With our program, you can use the motivation of better-quality sex for doing these exercises. There's nothing wrong with being very up-front and direct about it. But I suspect that, once started, you'll quickly find other motivators. Including just plain, pure, unadulterated enjoyment.

Motivation, however, is a rather strange critter. It needs to be constantly replenished or it exhausts itself. And if you have not previously engaged in a strenuous exercise program, don't make the mistake of telling yourself you can't do it because you don't have the motivation of so-and-so, who religiously follows an exercising program every single day. Even the most ardent exerciser

has days when it is a chore to get down and do it.

Failing to have motivation is only human. Motivation resulting from a desire to improve is, however, a very human trait. Animals are motivated by simple things like hunger, fear, sex. They cannot look into the future and say, "If I walk from here to the next town today, it'll make me stronger and more able to do a better job of it next week." But human beings can look down the road and see a goal they want to reach, and they can then motivate themselves to try to attain that goal.

If you want well-toned muscles or to improve your sex life, you can bring into effect certain factors that will help you attain those goals. The goal at the end of the effort is the thing that fuels the motivation, and the motivation applied to your daily life is what brings about the way to that goal.

There are many ways you can motivate yourself. I know two people who are motivated by a painting they saw in a magazine. They tore the page from the magazine and attached it to their refrigerator door; the painting is of two very old people, complete with a lifetime of wrinkles on their faces. They are smiling at whoever happens to pass by, as they contemplate their exercising routine; they are wearing tight-fitting sweat suits, and their bodies are like those of twenty-five-year-olds. These two people I know look at that picture every time they go to raid the refrigerator for a snack, and they pass it on their way out the door to go on a run. "It's kind of a long-, long-term goal, but old age won't be half-bad if you can keep moving through it under your own head of steam," they'll tell anyone who asks about the picture. They've got a good point.

Find something to motivate yourself. And your best bet to provide that motivation is *YOU*. Do it for yourself. Don't be overwhelmed by exercises. You're your own worst obstacle. Too many people look at others exercising and let themselves be overwhelmed. They see exercise as one mountain of a challenge. They make the mistake of not breaking exercise down into its components. Break it down, and exercising is as easy or as difficult as you can make it.

So many women tell me that exercising is too much for them, that they know they can't do this or that exercise. And because they know they can't do certain exercises, they back away from exercising altogether. There are some exercises that I can't do. And there are some exercises that I can do — but only if I've faithfully kept to my regular program. For some exercises; you must have your body perfectly toned and flexible. And there are some exercises that some people will never be able to do.

On the other hand, there are many exercises that you might not be able to do right now, yet regularly working at simpler exercises prepares your body for the more difficult ones. Exercising, like everything else, is a gradual growth process.

If you really want to convince yourself that you can do an exercise, go to a gym or health spa and watch someone who is very good at exercising. But be sure to get there before the exerciser starts her workout. Notice that the exerciser begins with extremely simple moves. They are exercises that you would have little trouble doing. She does them for two reasons:

1. Exercising at high levels is based on a foundation of exercising on a simple level.

2. Even the most advanced exerciser starts and ends a routine with simple exercises, because they are used to warm up and then to cool down the body, an essential part of exercising. You'll never see an experienced exerciser jump right into a difficult exercise. The body must first be warmed up, and it is warmed up by simple, basic exercises. The routine, if graphed according to effort, would depict a bell-shaped curve. The routine starts out easy, to warm the body; it becomes gradually more difficult; then it peaks with the most difficult exercises. Finally, the exercises get easier and the routine ends with simple exercises.

In other words, you don't climb the mountain until you've been in the pits. The pits. The trenches. The simplistic. Whatever you call it, you can forget the negative connotations. If I'm pressed for time to fit a workout into my day, it may just consist of a dozen very simple, basic exercises. Just enough to keep my body loose, and my routine intact — not that I'm going to die if I miss a day. I don't need that kind of pressure on myself.

I try to do at least some exercising every day, but once in a while I'll miss a day. When I have the time, I like to do a long workout, and not all of it is difficult. So what's the bottom line? There is really no ex-cuse not to begin an exercise program, which will give you the capacity to engage in more fulfilling, enjoyable lovemaking.

Sweating doesn't make you less of a lady; in fact, it can give you a very natural and genuine blush of youth, which you can't get from cosmetics.

The hang-ups about those terrible calisthenics in high-school PE classes can be overcome. You were forced to do them then; now they're under control.

As for motivation, that's up to you. The rewards are legion: more fulfilling sex; trim, slim body; the ability to move through life with grace and forcefulness; the ability to keep it up longer and more often. Your personal needs and desires provide your motivation.

Still thinking exercises are too difficult and that you can't do them? Well, you don't get your driving permit one day and race at the Indianapolis 500 the next. And you don't decide on an exercise program today, and twist yourself into a pretzel tomorrow. You start with the Casual Level Sexercises, move through them one at a time, adding exercises as your progress, and build from there.

Just a few words about getting yourself set to start. There is no special equipment needed for these exercises. They all can be done at home, at your local health spa, in the living room with friends, even in the family room. I occasionally exercise with some friends or take an exercise class — as much to be with other people having similar interests as in an attempt to learn new exercising techniques. But I also like to exercise alone periodically.

I'm also fond of exercising to music, which I pick to fit my mood. (There is a separate chapter on matching certain exercise sequences with specific music, but what I'm referring to here is mood music, something conducive to exercise by.)

Keep a throw rug handy if you must exercise on a hardwood floor. Avoid drafty areas to exercise in, because cold air causes muscles to tighten. As for clothing, wear what you feel most comfortable in when you are exercising.

If you are just starting an exercise program, I don't advise going out to purchase a lot of expensive clothing. Start with what you have around the house; as you get more into exercising, check out clothing that might be more comfortable to work out in.

Go ahead and use your old gym clothes at first, if you saved them and they still fit. You can put off the leg-warmers and all the other "status" apparel until you are ready to take an exercise class, where showing off is part of the game.

Keep your exercises simple and streamlined. Complicated exercises will only make exercising a chore.

The time of day you do the exercises is entirely up to you. Some people like to exercise first-thing in the morning; others find it most convenient at lunchtime, thereby neatly breaking up the day into two segments; still others like to exercise before the evening meal. They might feel that they're loose then, making exercise more comfortable, and that a workout invigorates them for the evening ahead. It is often pleasant to exercise for an hour, take a shower, and then get dressed for a night on the town; the exercise gets your blood pumping and clears out the fatigue from a busy day. You'll be more alert, ready for anything that night.

Do your exercising when it suits you — and your body. The more relaxed you are when you exercise, the less likely you are to experience discomfort or to strain something. So try to work your exercising in with your body's schedule for the day. Make the time of your workout a habit. If you find it is best to exercise at five in the evening, schedule your plans around that. Exercising can quickly become a daily routine, like brushing your teeth.

Now remember, the exercises in this chapter are not only for novice exercisers, but also can be used as warmups or cooldowns for more experienced exercisers. This chapter, then, should be the one most used in the book. Fifty exercises are presented here. You're *not* expected to do them all at one time. Do as many as *you* feel comfortable with. Add one or two as you feel like it.

Each exercise is described, and features a photo-sequence of how I do the exercise. The part or parts of the body the exercise affects *most* are described. Obviously, an exercise may affect other parts of the body than the ones mentioned. Following is an illustration of one or more sexual positions that would benefit from a regular and faithful use of this exercise. You may be unfamiliar with some of these sexual positions. If so, you might want to give them a try.

Okay. Let's get to it. Roll out that rug, turn on that music, put a smile on your face, and in your heart, and put that body through its paces.

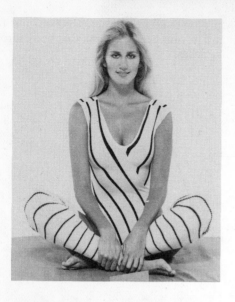

HEAD ROLL

This is excellent for those times when you've developed a lot of tension from your hectic day. The Head Roll is very easy to do, and can even be done at the office or in your home. Merely close the door for a few moments and sit down. Sitting cross-legged on the floor, close your eyes and drop your chin to your chest. Concentrate on relaxing totally. Gravity will pull your head down, stretching the muscles in the back of the neck. When you are completely relaxed, roll your head clockwise. Roll it in a circle around your shoulders, pretending it is not connected. Do this ten times in the clockwise direction, pause, then reverse and do it counterclockwise.

Benefits: Excellent for relieving tension in the neck and shoulders.

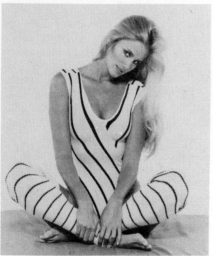

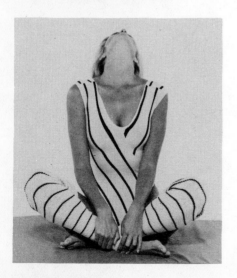

ACHILLES SAVER

If you are active in sports, or if you get heavily into your Sexercises, your Achilles tendon, which connects the lower calf with the back of the heel, will get quite a workout. To prevent injury to it, the tendon must be stretched periodically. Stretching keeps it pliable and supple; a tight Achilles has a greater chance of being injured. There is a very simple Sexercise you can do to save your Achilles tendon a lot of grief. (Oh, yes, wearing high-heels causes tight Achilles, and this Sexercise is perfect for keeping your Achilles healthy and happy.) Use any object that will serve as a step. Walk up to the object or step and step up onto it. Now, slowly and carefully back both feet off the step, until you have only the front one-third of your feet still on the step or raised platform. For balance, do this next to a wall or banister so you can support yourself on it. Now, keeping your legs straight and together, lower your heels, bending the feet slightly. You should feel the Achilles tendons stretching. When the stretch becomes slightly uncomfortable, stop and hold for a count of five. Bring your feet back up, pause for a moment, and then lower your heels again, this time holding for a count of seven. Return. Lower yourself again for a count of ten. Return. Lower for a count of twelve. Return. Lower for a count of five. Return. Now, walk around for a minute or until your muscles and tendons feel back into balance.

Benefits: Stretches Achilles tendon, and helps prevent tightness and tendon injuries.

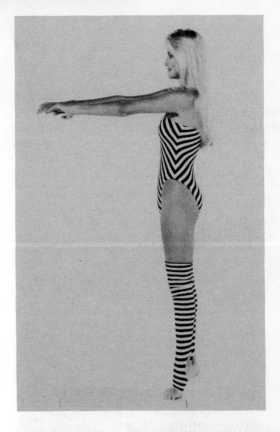

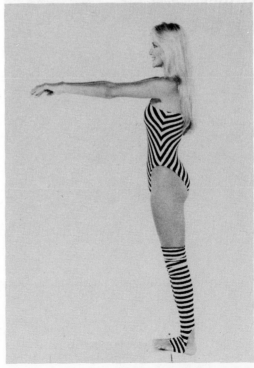

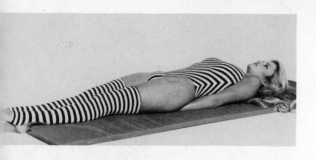

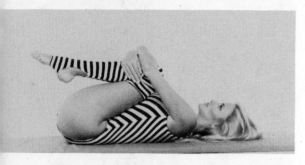

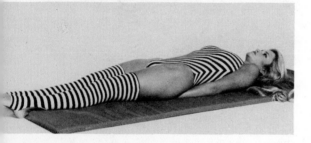

DOUBLE TUCK

This one is extremely simple, and you've probably done it yourself as a kid. First lie down on the floor on your back. Bring your bent knees up to your chest as far as you can. Now, wrap your arms around your legs and pull your legs even tighter to your chest. Hold for twenty seconds, and release. Repeat five times.

Variation: You can do the same Sexercise one leg at a time, extending the straight leg to its maximum length.

Benefits: Terrific for flexibility in the back of the legs and in the lower back.

THE FELINE STRETCH

In yoga circles, this one is referred to simply as "The Cat." It is an exercise that particularly benefits back flexibility and builds leg and arm strength. For the female, the sexual positions possible from The Feline Stretch are fairly obvious. You can enjoy this Sexercise merely for its luxurious aspects. Let yourself go and you'll soon realize what kind of exquisite feelings a cat gets when it stretches itself after a nap. Get down on your hands and knees. Now, keeping your palms planted on the floor, in one sensuous and continuous motion drop your head toward your hands (keeping your arms straight), while arching your back. Use the shoulders and hips as hinges. Reach for the ceiling with the middle of your back. Hold it there for two seconds. Then, in the same smooth and sensuous movement, bring your head up and your back down, keeping shoulders and hips stationary. Try to reach the floor with your tummy. Feel your muscles stretch themselves luxuriously. Return to the starting position, and repeat The Feline Stretch twenty times.

Benefits: Strengthens arms and thighs, and increases flexibility in the lower back and neck.

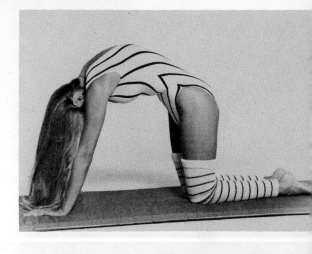

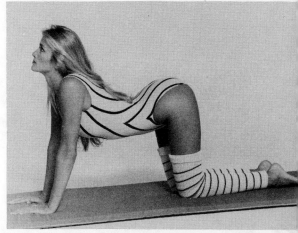

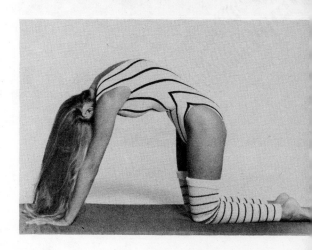

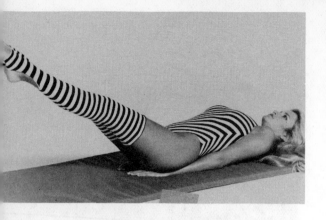

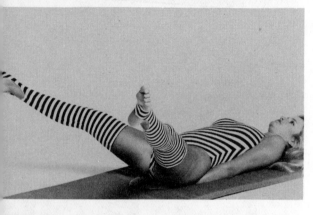

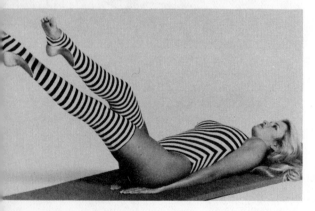

THE SILK CROSSOVER

The female legs are the most used and stressed parts of her anatomy during intercourse. She must spread them for sometimes unendurable amounts of time. They must therefore be as strong and as flexible as possible. For men, developing leg flexibility and strength can go a long way in going a long way. Start The Silk Crossover by lying on your back, with your hands under your buttocks, palms on the floor. Now, the only body parts you want to move are your legs, and you want to keep them perfectly straight when you do move them. Bring your legs up to a 45-degree angle, keeping them straight and together. Now, spread them as wide as they'll go, hold for a count of five, and then bring them back toward each other. But instead of joining them again, pass the right leg over the left until you meet resistance along your thighs. Then, in one smooth motion, bring them back to a spread position, hold for a count of five, and return them. This time you pass your left leg over your right, again until you meet resistance. Repeat The Silk Crossover thirty times, each time alternating which leg passes over the other.

Benefits: Strengthens the thighs and inner thighs, and increases flexibility; also tones and smooths the inner thighs.

CYCLE SAVAGES

Cycle Savages are fun, and I'll bet that you did them as a kid. And you can still be terrific at doing them. They are the inverted bicycle, or riding-the-bike. Start by lying on your back; then, tuck your legs together and bring them toward your chest, continuing to roll until they are over your head and you are touching the floor with only your shoulders and the back of your head. Support your legs by placing your hands on your waist and putting your elbows on the floor. Now, as you are reading, begin pumping your legs in a circular fashion, just as if you were riding a bicycle. Don't pump furiously or you'll tire yourself out too quickly. Start slowly and build your speed as you get rolling. Do this one for as long as you can — until your legs begin to feel wobbly. Then come out of the position and rest for about sixty seconds, allowing the blood to flow back into your lower extremities.

Benefits: Increases sense of balance and builds leg strength and leg speed.

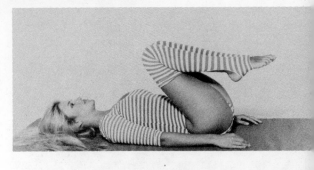

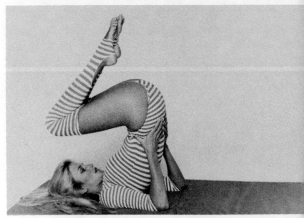

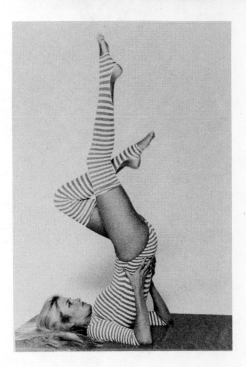

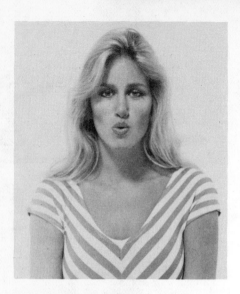

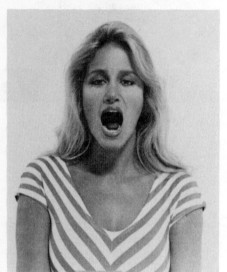

OOHHS & AAHHS

This can be done before or after the Tongue Lashes, and is used to strengthen the mouth. Continue sitting down or lying down, and with the rest of your body relaxed, concentrate on your lips. Very elaborately, form the shape you make with your lips when you say "Oooooh" and hold it for about ten seconds; then go right into opening your mouth as wide as it will go by saying "Aaaaah" for ten seconds. Now go back to the "Oooooh" and then the "Aaaaah." Do each ten times.

Benefits: Strengthens lips and mouth.

TONGUE LASHES

Go ahead and laugh. It does seem pretty funny — until you realize that the only exercising your tongue gets is while moving around food when you're eating, and moving about in the mouth while you talk. From a Sexercise standard, think about how important the tongue is — and how it deserves strengthening just as other muscles. See, that's the difference between just-plain-exercising and Sexercising. You can do this one before, after, or during pauses in exercise routines. Sit on the floor, perhaps in the lotus position; or, you can lie on your back. The tongue can move through just about any plane you wish. Now, stick your tongue out as far as it will go, and do the following six Sexercises with it: 1. Spin it ten times clockwise, then reverse and spin it ten times counterclockwise. 2. Make X's and crosses (the religious type) with your tongue, ten times each. 3. Make five attempts to touch your nose with your tongue, and if you're successful all five times, send me your name and address. 4. Touch your chin with your tongue five times, or at least get as close as possible. 5. Spell your name with your tongue; you could do this on a pane of glass if you wanted to, or on a pocket mirror; be sure to clean it off afterward, however. 6. Flick your tongue side to side as fast as you can for fifteen seconds. Now give your tongue a rest, until it's needed when you meet your lover.

Benefits: Builds flexibility, extension and strength in the tongue.

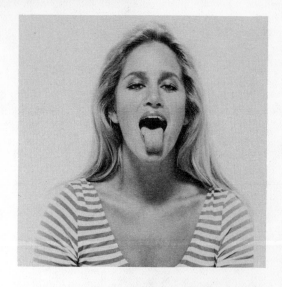

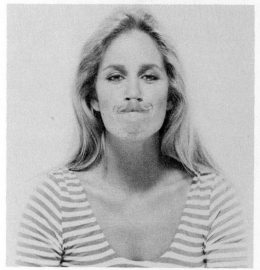

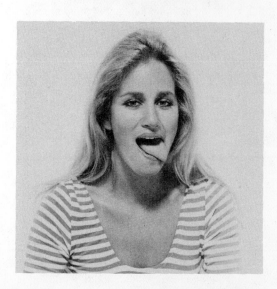

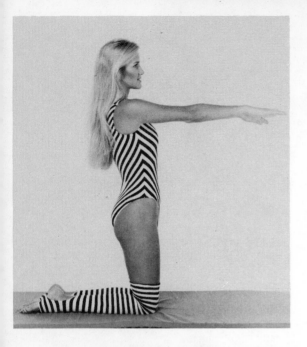

THE LONG RIDE

A good lovemaking session is often wilted by one or the other of the partners tiring prematurely. At least that's true for those who go in for more than a wham-bam-thank-you-mam approach to lovemaking. An exhausting session leaves you feeling like a marathon runner who is totally wasted in the latter stages of a race. One of the first parts to go, at about eighteen miles, is the front, upper leg. The Long Ride exercise is excellent for improving muscle strength in the front thigh and should be appreciated by marathoners, and by lovers who like to take that long ride. This is great for females who like to get on top in lovemaking, and for males who like to make a rear entrance. Start by kneeling on the floor, back military-straight. Reach your arms out in front of you so they stay parallel to the floor. Now slowly lean back until you feel a pull on your thighs. Keep everything from the back of the knees to the back of the head perfectly straight so that the body leans back as one unit. Lean back until the pull on your legs is on the verge of discomfort, and then hold for a count of five. Return to the upright position, take a short breath, and then repeat twenty times. After a few weeks, you should notice distinct improvements in your ability to go for the long one.

Benefits: Strengthens the front of the upper legs and lower back muscles.

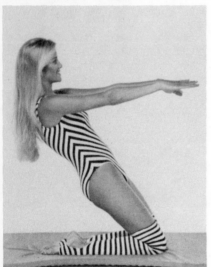

THE LONG ARCH

The Long Arch takes The Long Ride just a few steps farther. Kneel down on the floor, and place your hands on your hips. Bend backward slowly, keeping your back straight and making all movements controlled and deliberate. Do not rush this one. You will experience a pulling sensation in your thighs and through the front of your body. The object is to lie back and touch your head to the floor, behind your feet. Don't expect that you should be able to do this on the first try. As with the Stationary Butterfly, allow gravity to help you with The Long Arch. If you have any sort of back problems, be very careful. Many people I know, both men and women, find that this workout gives them an incredible amount of flexibility in the front of the body, although many of them said on their first attempts they had a great deal of trouble getting themselves back up once they had gone down. If you can't bring yourself back up on the strength of your abdominals, use your hands, or roll over onto your side before doing the Long Arch again. When you have this one down, plan on resting for about a minute before coming back up. Do this one five times.

Benefits: Increases strength in the thighs and the abdominal muscles, while also increasing the flexibility in the front torso.

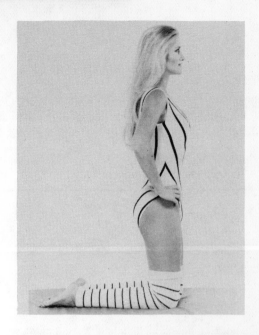

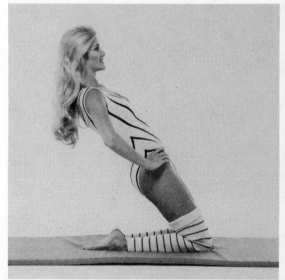

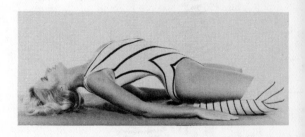

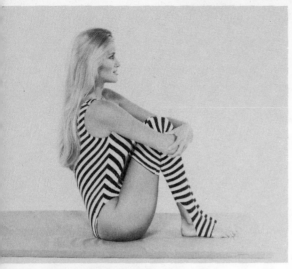

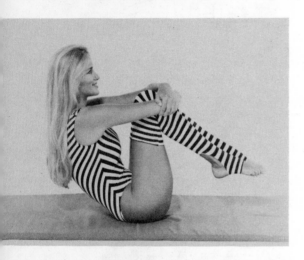

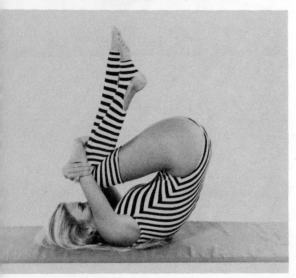

THE SOWBUG

This one harkens back to when you were a child. Sit on the floor and pull your legs up to your chest as far as they'll go. Now, wrap your arms around your legs and pull your legs even closer to you. Give a little push-off with your toes and roll backward onto your back. Keep rolling back until the back of your neck stops you. Don't bang your head, though. When you reach that point, roll forward again. Roll forward and backward ten times.

Benefits: Terrific stretch for the spine.

THE TURTLE

This is a good stretching Sexercise to throw in between difficult sequences. Kneel down on the floor, resting your buttocks on your heels. Now, stretch out your arms in front of you and bend forward from the hips. Tuck your head down between your outstretched arms. Allow gravity to pull you down into a curled-up ball. Hold this position for as long as you like. To make the stretch even more effective, allow your fingers to pull you forward by slowly, inch by inch, pulling them along the floor.

Benefits: Excellent stretch for the upper body.

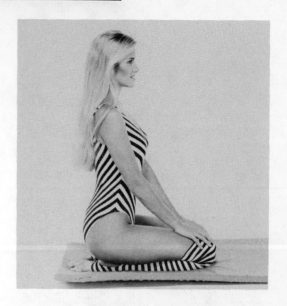

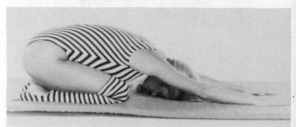

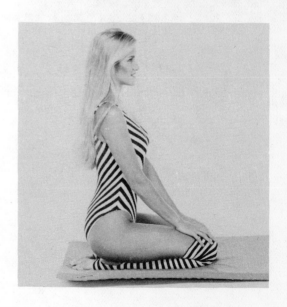

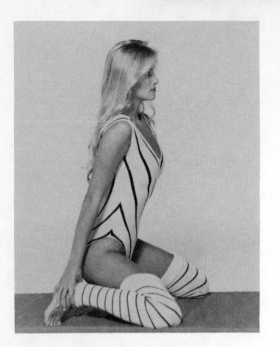

THE SQUATTER

Go into a squat and slowly lower your knees to the floor. Keep your toes dug into the carpet or floor, because that's the fulcrum of your balancing act. Now, keeping your back straight, reach around on both sides and plant your palms on your heels, making sure that the arms stay straight. Here comes the hard part. Without removing your hands from your heels, and keeping your back and your arms straight, roll back onto your soles. Your roll should take you into a flat-footed squat, almost as if you were Harry Houdini himself, rolling into a ball to be placed in a box. Now, go back up onto your toes and from there back to your knees. Repeat the move ten times.

Benefits: Tightens the buttocks, increases sense of balance and strengthens the back.

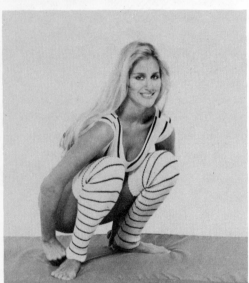

THE STAKE

Do you remember in the old cowboy movies, where the hero would be captured by Indians and staked, spread-eagled, out in the desert sun? As the wet rawhide holding him dried, he'd get stretched. From doing those movies, that's how many of the cowboy heroes got to be as tall as they were, I'll bet. Well, this Sexercise isn't as terrible as all that. You have your hands free. The cowboy heroes always managed to free themselves anyway. Pretend that you're staked out in the desert, but you've got your hands free. So, start by spreading your legs in front of you in a 90-degree angle as you sit on the floor. Keep your back straight and sit up straight. Now, put your hands up over your head — arms straight, hands together. Keeping your legs, arms and back straight, and doing all the bending in the waist, touch your hands to your left foot (or as close to your foot as you can get), and then come back up to your original position. Then do the same thing to your right foot, returning to your original position. Repeat The Stake fifteen times to each side.

Benefits: Great for flexibility in the back and the back of the legs, and excellent for stretching the inner thighs.

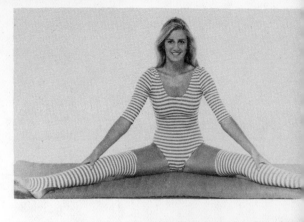

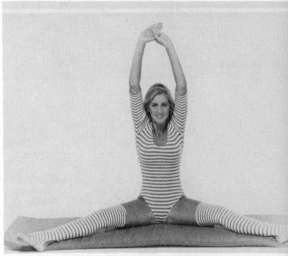

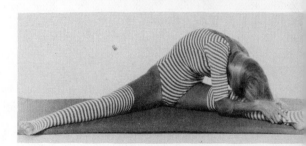

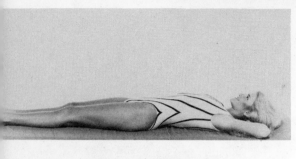

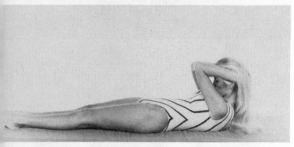

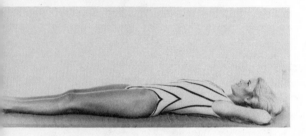

NECKER

This one is incredibly simple, but very, very effective. Lie down on your back, legs straight but relaxed. Now, clasp your hands behind your neck and pull your head forward until your chin touches your chest. Hold for five seconds and return your head to the floor. Repeat this one ten times. Later, as you build strength in your neck, do the same exercise without using your hands, and slowly increase the amount of time you hold your chin to your chest.

Benefits: Terrific for building strength in the neck muscles.

THE SPHINX

Start this one by lying on the floor, as though you were going to do a push-up. Place your hands at shoulder-width in the push-up position, but instead of keeping your legs together behind you, spread them wide apart. Now, keeping your legs on the floor, push your upper body off the floor, arching the back and throwing back the head; keep your hips on the floor. It you have any back problems, be very careful in doing this one; only push up to the point of discomfort, and then stop. Don't overdo it. Holding your position, bring your feet together (bend your legs at the knees) behind your head, bringing them as close to your head as is possible. Hold your position for a count of five, and then smoothly return to the starting position. Repeat this one five times.

Benefits: Builds flexibility in the lower back and legs, and strength in the arms.

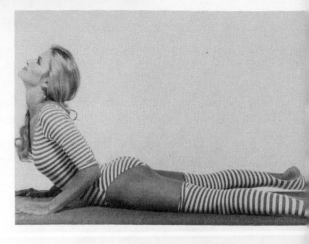

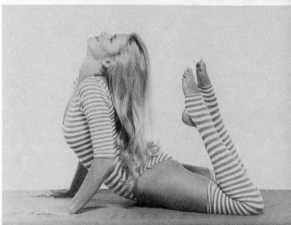

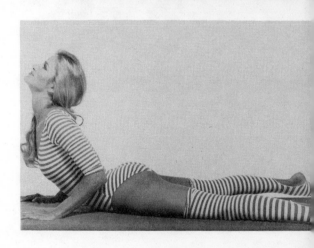

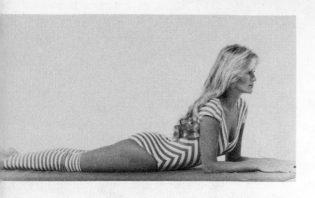

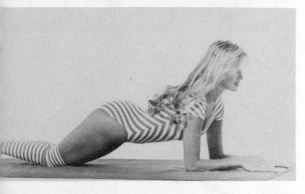

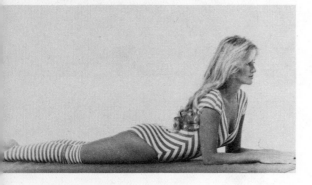

SPHINX DROP

Get down on the floor on your stomach. Support yourself with your palms, forearms and elbows positioned flat on the floor and in front of you; you are posing very much like the Sphinx in Egypt. Keep the entire front of your body immobile for this exercise. Only the part of your body between the elbows and knees — your torso — should move. Lift the pelvic area and make rapid movements up and down, just as you and your partner do during lovemaking. Keep the motion fluid. Repeat twenty times. Now, as a variation, twist your hips while they are in the "up" position.

Benefits: Builds strength and flexibility in the hips.

SUPER TOUCH

This is a delightful combination of Superman in flight and the standard toe-touch. It is one that, if you close your eyes while doing the upper portion of it, you can really get off on. Begin by standing straight, legs together, hands on hips. Then, in one fluid motion, as though you were diving or flying through the air like Superman, reach for the sky and go up on your toes. When you have extended to your maximum, come back to the original position with hands on hips; then, continuing the motion, go down into a toe-touch, keeping the legs straight and bending at the hips. If you can't touch your toes at first, go as far as the limits of comfort, and keep working on it. As you get better and become more flexible, you'll be able to do a toe-touch. Repeat this one twenty times.

Benefits: Stretches legs and arms; builds flexibility in hips.

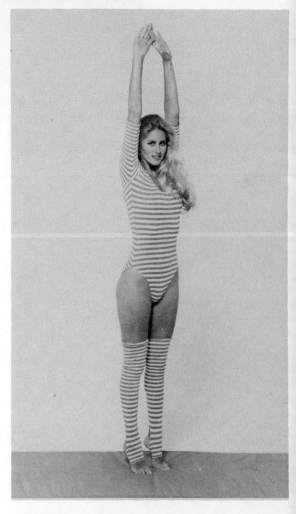

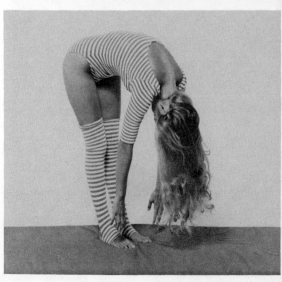

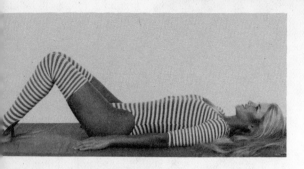

PELVIC PUNCH

This one is easy and it's a lot of fun; it also benefits the all-important pelvic area. Lie on your back. Keep your legs straight and together. Now, place your arms along your sides. Bend your knees slightly — just enough so that you can place the soles of your feet flat on the floor. Now, raise your buttocks about four inches off the floor, lifting at the waist. Raise the pelvis toward the ceiling, and then bring it back to four inches off the floor, where you started. Use a smooth, rhythmic motion. Get the picture? This should be done about fifteen times; then lower your buttocks on the floor, take a breath and repeat another fifteen times.

Benefits: Adds flexibility to the pelvic area, while strengthening the thighs and buttocks.

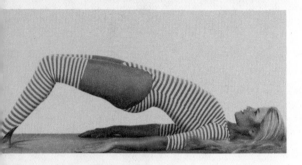

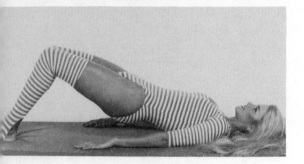

PELVIC WAVE

This one is similar to the Pelvic Punch, but instead of an up-and-down motion, you use a back-and-forth motion. Start by lying on your back, legs out straight and together. Place your arms next to your sides. Bend your legs at the knees just enough so you can place the soles of your feet flat on the floor. Now, raise your buttocks about four inches off the floor, and begin swinging your pelvis back and forth as though it were a porch swing. Do this swing fifteen times, then lower yourself for a short rest, and repeat fifteen times more.

Benefits: Strengthens the thighs and provides flexibility to the hips and pelvic area.

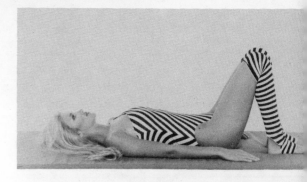

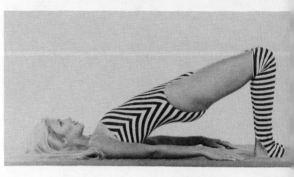

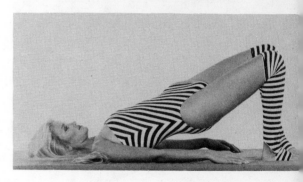

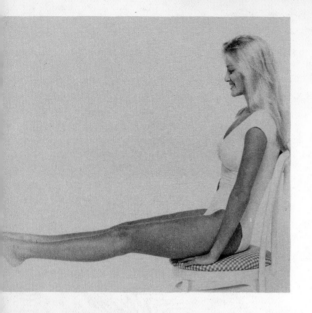

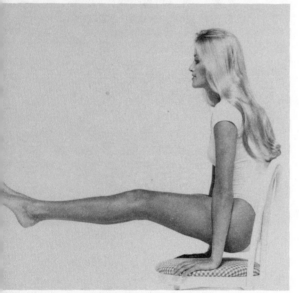

THE PELVIC LIFT

This one is great for the arms and for the body control in the hips. Sit on the edge of a bed or a heavy chair. Place your hands down on the bed or chair seat, next to your hips. Raise your legs out in front of you, keeping them together and straight. Lift yourself off the seat by pushing up with your hands. This takes considerable strength in the arms, and requires balance in the hips. Don't be concerned if you can't push yourself completely off the chair at first. If you get your pelvic area up and the backs of your legs are still in contact with the chair, that's a start. The object is to build strength in the arms and body awareness in the hips and legs. Once you get it down, though, try to hold it for fifteen seconds, and repeat it five times.

Benefits: Builds strength in the arms and pelvic area, while increasing flexibility and body awareness in the pelvic area.

THE ROTATION

Your waist and hips will get a workout from this one, both in building strength and flexibility. Begin by standing up straight, with your hands on your hips. Now, spread your feet as wide as your shoulders, to provide a base of support. The object is to rotate your upper body on the axis of your hips, while keeping the legs and buttocks stationary. Start by bending forward at the waist, your hands still on your hips. When your upper body is still parallel to the floor, slowly rotate your entire body to the right. Continue through and rotate on the hips to the back, across the back, and into the left. Finish up in the starting position, having done a complete 360-degree circle. This is going to be a bit awkward at first, because you are not going to be perfectly flexible and, of course, you cannot force your back to go into a position it was never built for, which would be bending back until it is parallel to floor on the rear-most extension. Do The Rotation slowly and completely under control. Do it ten times in the direction to the right, stop a moment, and then reverse it for ten more rotations.

Benefits: Builds flexibility in the hips and waist, and stretches the abdomen, back and sides.

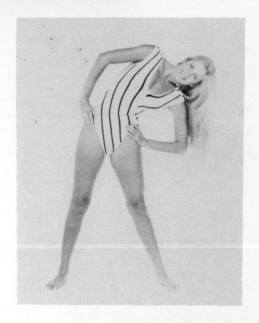

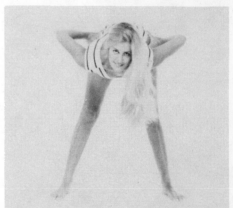

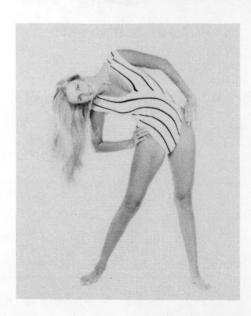

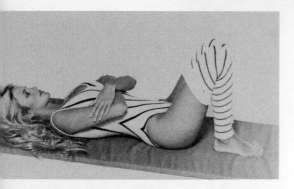

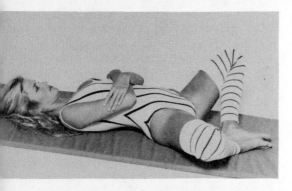

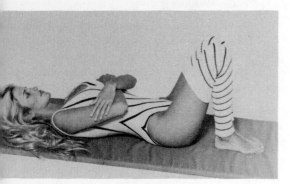

STATIONARY BUTTERFLY

This one is extremely easy, because you allow gravity to do all of your work for you. Lie on your back, and cross your arms on your chest — you won't be needing them. Now, bend your legs at the knees, keeping them together, your heels just about touching your buttocks. Allowing gravity to do its thing, let your legs fall to the sides, thus bringing your soles together. It is unlikely that you will be so flexible that your legs will actually make contact with the floor, but that is the goal. Do not force anything. Just lie there resting, allowing gravity to bring your legs toward the floor. You should feel mild stretching in the groin area and along the inner thighs. Do this for about a minute, or as long as it is still comfortable, then return to your original position, with your legs bent but together. Then, stretch your legs out as though you were standing erect. This position will allow your legs to relax from the groin stretch. Then return to the bent-knee position, and let gravity go to work. The Stationary Butterfly is very passive, but very effective. Repeat this one five times as a loosening-up exercise.

Benefits: Adds flexibility to the groin area and stretches the inner thigh area.

THE STARGAZER

This one is great for keeping the insides of the thighs supple. Stand up straight. Now, take a step forward; leave your trailing leg planted on the floor, and keep it straight. Bend the leading leg at the knee, while placing your hands on the thigh, above the knee. Then, lean your head back until you are gazing directly at the ceiling. Hold that position for a count of five, keeping your back straight. Next, stand up straight, keeping your hands together in front of you. You will not switch legs. Assume the same position as before, but now you should be working the opposite leg. Keep the heel of the trailing leg planted on the floor, and your Achilles tendon will get a good stretch. Do The Stargazer five times to start, and eventually increase to twenty times.

Benefits: Stretches the Achilles tendon and builds strength in the thighs.

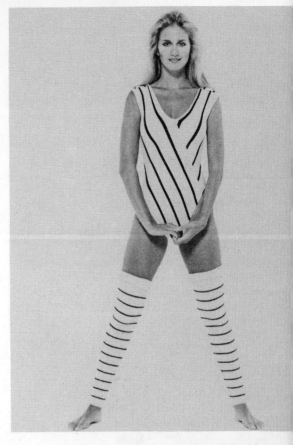

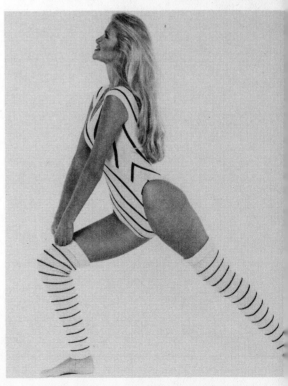

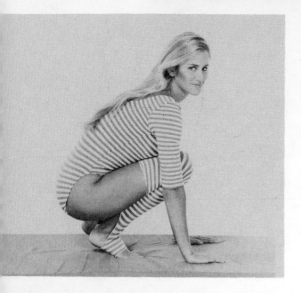

THE SPRINTER

This is an Olympic event for you to practice in order to get that world-class style for your serious encounters. You'll do an exaggerated version of a sprinter's crouch in this exercise. Crouch down, placing your hands in front of you on the floor. Now, extend your left leg behind you. Stretch it out until it is completely straight. The more strain you can put on the foot of the extended leg, the better stretch you'll get for the backs of the legs and the groin area. Hold this pose for fifteen seconds, and then return to the neutral crouch. Take a breath, and then extend the other leg. While your trailing leg is extended, you can stretch the muscles in that leg by putting more or less weight on the trailing foot. You should be able to feel the difference. This makes you conscious of where your leg muscles connect. This exercise is particularly good for stretching leg muscles that you will use in wide-open sex positions. Do The Sprinter ten times in each leg.

Benefits: Tremendous benefits to the Achilles tendon, hamstring and lower back.

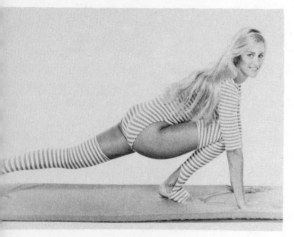

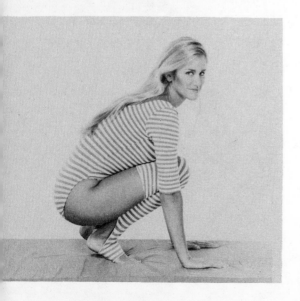

THE HURDLER

You can have dreams of Olympic glory with this one. You'll be able to twist yourself into shape for some terrific performances at home, too. Start by sitting on the floor. Extend one leg out in front of you, and tuck the other one under you; the heel of the foot of your tucked leg should be against your buttocks. Reach for your extended foot with both arms and pull your forehead down to your kneecap very slowly. Ease back to the starting position. Now, lean back and let gravity pull your body toward the floor behind you, until your back rests against the floor. Pause, count to three, and slowly return to your neutral, upright position. If at first you cannot lean all the way down, be patient; go down as far as you comfortably can, and keep working at it until you can easily imagine yourself lightly brushing the top of the hurdle on your way to breaking the tape. Do this one five times.

Benefits: Adds tremendous flexibility to the hips, pelvis and legs; builds strength in the abdomen and back.

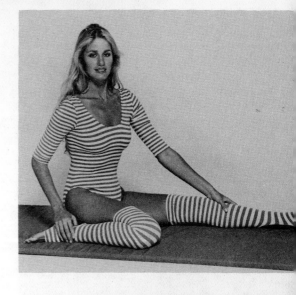

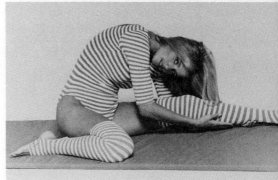

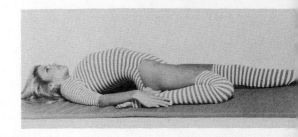

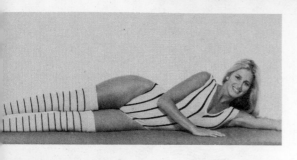

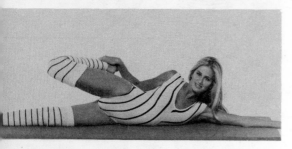

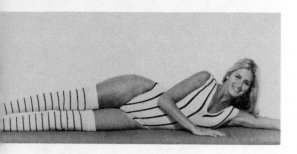

SIDE HURDLER

Begin by lying down on your right side. Extend your right arm out along the floor so that a straight line could be drawn from your right hand to your feet. Now, with your left hand, grasp your left foot as you bend your left leg to bring it toward you. Once you have a good grasp, continue to pull, behind you now. Imagine yourself as an Olympic hurdler, just clearing the crossbar. Bring your left leg back as far as it will comfortably go, until it meets resistance. Hold for a count of ten in a relaxed mode, and then return to your original position. Repeat this one five times, and then roll to your left side and do it on the left side five times.

Benefits: Promotes flexibility in the quads and stretches the arms.

HURDLER COMPLEX

Sit down on the floor and tuck your right leg up and under you, with your heel touching your buttocks. Extend your left leg out in front of you, keeping it straight. Bend at the hips. While you are down here, reach forward and grasp your ankle with your hands. Using the hands, pull your body forward until you feel resistance. Then, moving at the hip, slowly return to an upright position and take a breath. Now, lean forward again, grasping your left foot with your right hand, while passing your left arm across your abdomen to grasp your tucked-in right leg. Using this new leverage, pull yourself forward, and again attempt to touch your nose to your left knee. Your head should be tucked under your right arm. Hold for a count of five, and return to the upright position. Repeat the Hurdler Complex five times with your left leg extended, switch and extend your right leg and repeat the exercise five more times.

Benefits: Excellent for stretching the legs, and adding flexibility and strength to the back and arms.

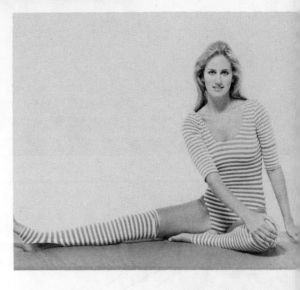

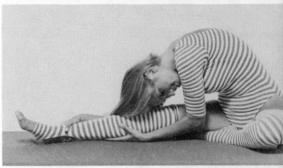

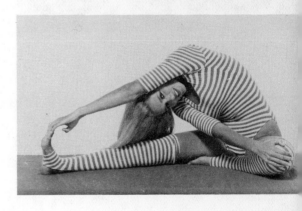

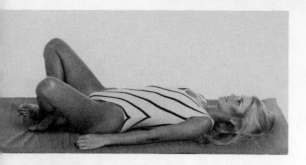

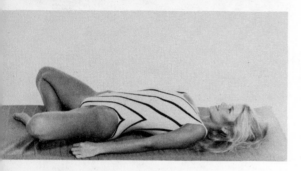

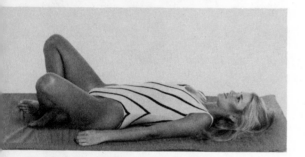

THE DOVE

Lie on your back. Bend your legs at the knees, and slide your feet to your buttocks, soles together. Now, flap your legs up and down until each leg touches the floor simultaneously, like the wings of a bird flapping on take-off. Be gentle at first, and as you warm up flap faster. The shoulders should be flat on the floor and all motion should be from hips on down. The Dove works the groin and waist area.

Benefits: Stretches and strengthens the groin and waist area, and strengthens the legs.

HOOF-TO-MOUTH

Begin by sitting on the floor. Stretch your legs out in front of you, holding them together. Now, keeping the legs straight, lean forward, and grasp with both hands the right ankle. Slowly and gently pull yourself back to a sitting position, bringing your leg along with you so that by the time you are sitting up straight, you have your straight leg in front of you and you can bring your ankle to your lips. Hold for a count of five, and then slowly and gently return it to the floor. While you are down there, grasp the left ankle and bring the leg up. Alternate legs on each return to the floor, and work each leg ten times. Do not panic if you cannot pull your leg all the way up to a vertical position the first time. This is one of those Sexercises where you can start gently and make progress virtually every day; stick with it. You'll eventually be able to bring your ankle to your lips.

Benefits: Excellent stretch for the groin, hamstring, calf and Achilles tendon.

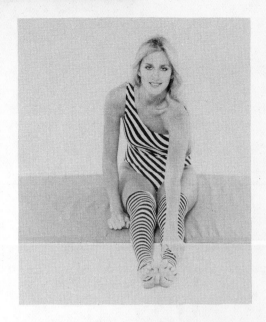

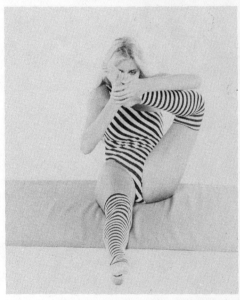

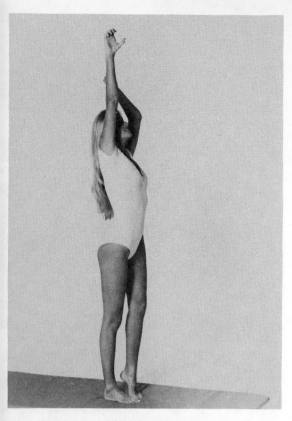

LADY APE

Here's where you get to allow your imagination to swing. Begin by standing up straight. Suck in your stomach. Now, tilt your head backward so that you are looking up. Bring your hands above your head and go through the motions of climbing a vine, as though you were climbing away from or toward Tarzan. Carry the climbing motion all the way down to your hips. Your motion should be sensuous and sinuous. Do Lady Ape for about three minutes. Finish by touching your toes and coming back to earth.

Benefits: Builds flexibility and strength in arms, and flexibility in the sides of the torso.

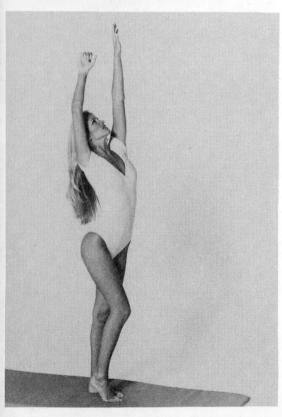

SKI SLOPE

Use your imagination while you are doing Ski Slope. Lie down on your back. Now, bending your legs at the knees, bring your heels as close to your buttocks as possible. Then lift your pelvis off the floor so that your thighs and trunk form a ski slope. Place your hands in the small of your back so that most of your body weight is supported by them; your elbows are in contact with the floor to complete the foundation. Hold the position for about twenty seconds and then relax. If you find your muscles having slight spasms while you are into the sixth or seventh of ten repetitions, just imagine that you are an earthquake happening on the ski slope, which isn't an impossibility in California. While you have your buttocks up in the air, tighten them.

Benefits: Excellent for warming up the back for an exercise session, and it also serves to strengthen the thighs and the buttocks.

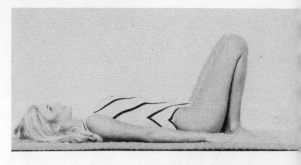

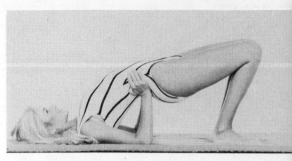

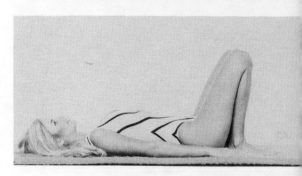

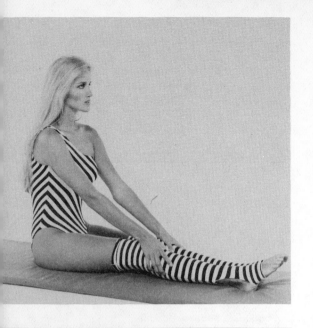

THE TRIANGLE

Sit down on the floor with both legs to-gether and extended in front of you. Keep them perfectly straight throughout the Sex-ercise. Now, in a very smooth motion, ex-tend your arms up over your head, bringing your hands together. Very slowly, and bend-ing at the waist, bow forward; the object is to grasp your feet with your hands. If you can, bend down far enough to touch your nose to your knees. If this is not possible, don't worry. It will come eventually. Hold the maximum extension of this Sexercise for a count of five, and then slowly return to your upright position. Repeat The Triangle five times when you start the Casual Level series, and ten times once you are regularly into the Intimate Level.

Benefits: Stretches muscles in the back and hamstrings.

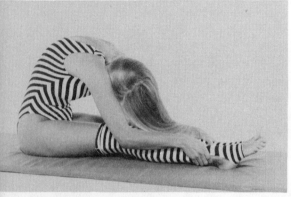

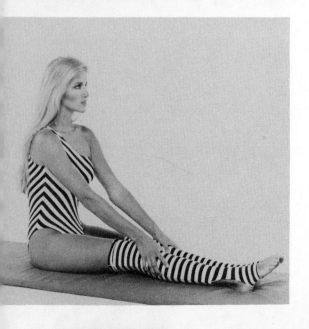

SWEEP WING

When you are doing Sweep Wing, think in terms of the supersonic jet fighters that feature the movable wings, which are swept back when the jet must reach high speeds. Pretend that you are the jet, sitting on the runway with your ground crew going through a pre-flight check. Get down on all fours. Now, extend your right leg straight out behind you. Keeping your entire leg parallel with and off the floor, swing the leg out to the side; move only at the hip joint, bringing the leg as far forward as you can, as though your leg were a jet wing. Repeat the forward thrust ten times; then return to your hands and knees, and repeat the same maneuver on the left leg.

Benefits: Terrific for strengthening the hip, pelvic region and waist.

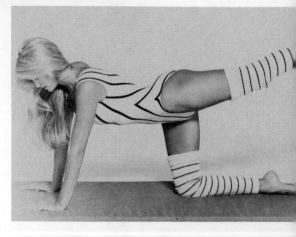

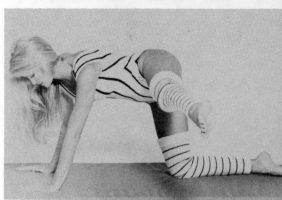

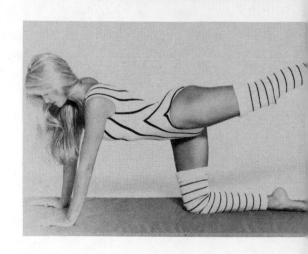

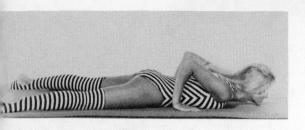

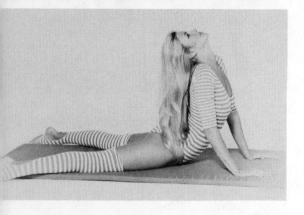

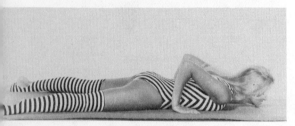

THE COBRA

In the film "*Black Stallion,*" a particularly memorable scene involved a snake. A boy and his jet-black horse were sleeping on the beach, as a cobra slithered down out of the sand. The cobra rose up in front of the young boy and extended its hood, ready to strike. Fortunately, the horse reacted in time to save the day. The cobra is one of the most deadly, but one of the most beautiful snakes in the world. There is a pose in yoga that honors the beautiful cobra, which works very well as a Sexercise. Start by lying on your stomach. Now, place the palms of your hands next to your waist, on the floor; cock your arms at the elbows to offer support. This exercise should not be performed if you have a weak back, because much of its benefit is centered on the back. Now, keeping your hips on the floor, raise your head as far off the floor as it will go, mimicking a cobra. Arch at your lower back, using your hands to give additional lift. When you achieve the maximum lift, tighten your buttocks and hold the pose for ten seconds before slowly dropping back to the floor. Your nose should eventually make contact with the floor; relax for a moment, and then repeat the exercise. Repeat The Cobra ten times.

Benefits: Builds strength in the lower back and stretches the front of the body.

LAZY FROG

Kneel down. Separate your knees about two feet and lower yourself through the gap. Try to be as pliable as you can, touching the floor. Don't point your toes outward while doing this, or you'll strain the knees; try to turn your toes inward, so that the tops of the feet are in contact with the floor. Now, in a very slow, deliberate and controlled manner, rotate your body up off the floor, into an upright position, doing all movement from the hips. Proceed to lean your back toward the floor. You can put your arms behind you for support so that you can lower yourself very, very slowly. This Sexercise is not recommended if you have back problems. When you reach the maximum backward tilt, relax there for a count of fifteen, and then slowly return to the starting position. If The Lazy Frog becomes especially easy for you, grab your ankles once you are down and gently pull them toward your body.

Benefits: Builds flexibility in the lower back and stretches the quads.

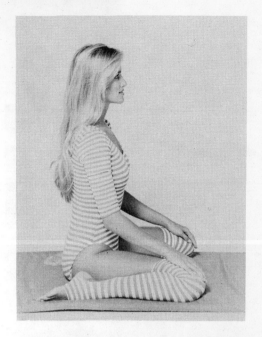

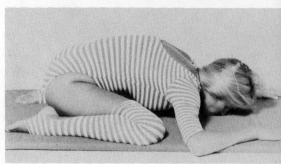

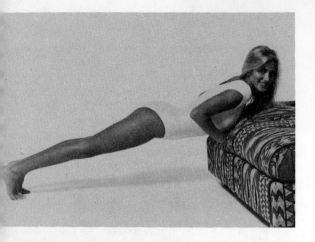

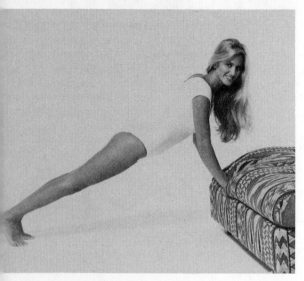

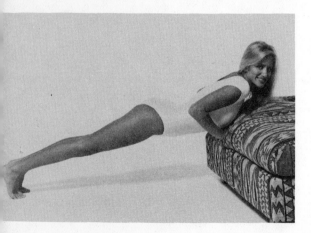

HALF PUSH-UPS

Not everyone has enough strength in her arms to do standard-issue push-ups. This applies to men as well. Anyone can build up to them, however; and everyone should, because strength in the arms is essential to good sex. Start at the bed, where your arms get some use. Kneel in front of your bed. Be sure that the bed is secure, so that it won't slide or roll when you start this workout. Bring your chest up against the bed, and palce your palms flat in front of you on the bed, shoulder-width apart. Now, take a breath and raise yourself on your arms, keeping your legs together. Then straighten the back and legs, so that you are in the standard push-up position, but your hands are on the edge of the bed. Go ahead and do some push-ups. You are building strength in your arms, but this is less difficult than a standard push-up because you do not have to bring your body all the way up from floor level. Repeat Half Push-Ups ten times.

Benefits: Builds strength in the arms and shoulders.

THE SWAY

Many women are bothered by lower-back pains. And for them, exercises stressing the lower back are certainly not recommended, except under the direction of their physicians. You can, however, build the lower back gradually in order to be able to return to normal activities, and this Sexercise (besides having obvious benefits for the male) is a fluid, smooth exercise for people needing just a bit of exercise on the lower back. Start by getting down on the floor as though you were going to do a standard push-up. Get up on the toes and keep the legs and back straight. But instead of flexing at the arms, dropping to the floor and then pushing yourself back up, drop the pelvis smoothly toward the floor, until your legs are parallel to the floor. As soon as your legs are parallel, however, bring them back up, keeping the motion fluid. The Sway should be repeated fifteen times.

Benefits: Builds strength in the arms and in the lower back, and builds flexibility in the spine.

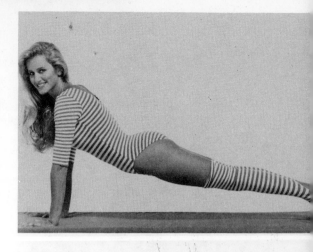

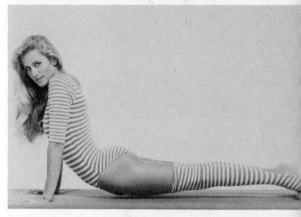

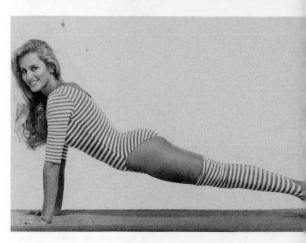

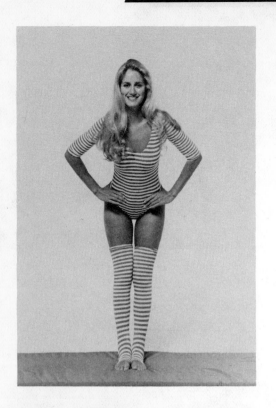

THE HIPPIE-HIPPIE SHAKE

This one looks deceptively simple, and once you've mastered it, it can be quite easy to do; you benefit from terrific flex in the pelvic region. Begin by standing with your hands on your hips, and your legs about two feet apart. You will use your hips only. Without moving your feet, and keeping your head and shoulders immobile, swivel your hips to the right, giving a gentle push with your left hand to get the machinery moving. As your hip reaches the extent of its extension to that side, swing it back around in a swiveling motion behind you, moving toward the left. The object is to keep the feet and head immobile while the hips swing around in a circular motion. If someone were looking down at you from above, he'd see your head in a perfectly stationary position, but below it the hips would be making a perfect circle. Do The Hippie-Hippie Shake for ten revolutions, then reverse direction for ten more twists.

Benefits: Increases flexibility in the hips and lower back.

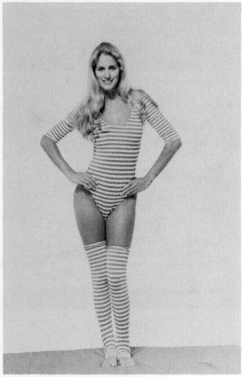

HOT-CROSS BUNS

This one is excellent for toning up the muscles on the hips and buns, and for adding a great deal of flexibility to the pelvic region. Start by sitting down on the floor, placing your hands behind you for support. Put your legs together and bend them at the knees. Now, being very careful not to move your arms or your head, and keeping your legs together, touch your left knee to the floor, making the rolling movement through the hips. Your heels should be up against your buttocks and your toes should keep contact with the floor. As soon as your knee touches, return to upright. Pause for a count of one, and then roll to the opposite side, touching the knee of the right leg to the floor, again keeping the head, arms and upper body straight, and the legs together. When you touch, return to the upright position. Repeat Hot-Cross Buns a total of ten times on each side.

Benefits: Tones the buns and adds flexibility to the pelvic region.

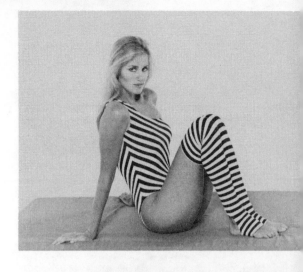

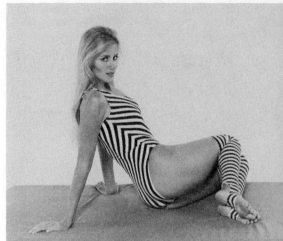

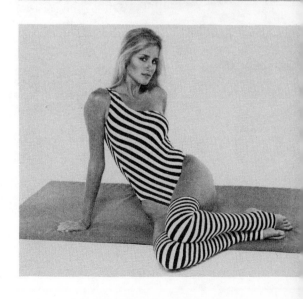

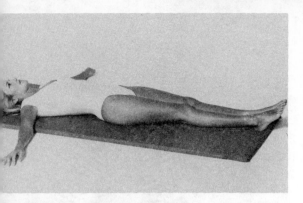

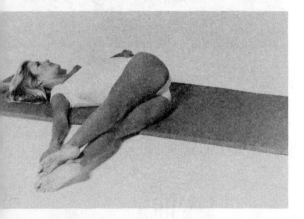

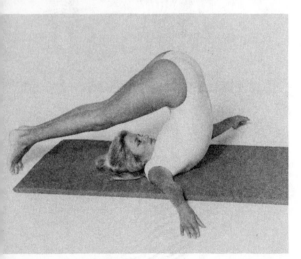

LEG ROLL

Start this one by lying down on the floor, on your back, legs together and straight. Now, for support, put your arms out perpendicular to your sides, palms down on the floor. Keeping your legs perfectly straight, roll them up to your hips, and attempt to bring your toes down just to the left of your chest, out in the area that constitutes the triangle formed by your side, your extended arm, and a line drawn from your fingers to your hip. If you can't touch the floor when you start, get your legs as near the floor as you can. Then, return your legs to their starting position, pause a moment, and bring them back up, keeping them straight and together, attempting to touch the floor behind your head. (So that you don't bash yourself in your nose with your knees, you can spread your legs about a foot as they approach your head.) When you touch or go as far as you can, return to the starting position, and pause. Then, bring your legs up again, and attempt to touch the floor in the triangle formed on your right side. Return to your starting position. Repeat the Leg Roll ten times. The mistake made most often in the Leg Roll is that people *try too hard,* making the legs tense. Try to remain calm and flexible.

Benefits: Terrific for the pelvic regions; loosens the hip joints, and builds the stomach muscles.

DOWN AND OUT

Stand straight with hands at your sides and ankles together. Now, very slowly and deliberately, settle down into a squat, making sure to keep the heels on the floor throughout. Once you are into the squat, separate your knees about a foot, and bring your hands together in front of you as though praying. Now, lower your arms down between your knees, locking your elbows up under your knees, right elbow to right knee, left elbow to left knee. Then, very gently, press outward against your legs with your elbows, spreading your legs even more. You can press your head down between your legs as you're doing this. The stretching that results should center on your groin area. Hold this position for thirty seconds, keeping the butt down as close to the floor as you can.

Benefits: Excellent stretch and warmup for the groin area.

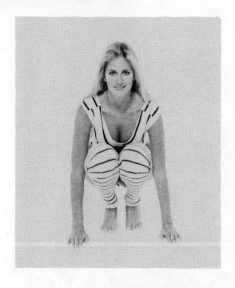

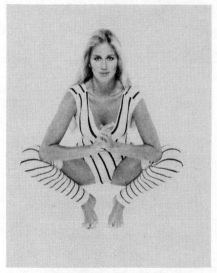

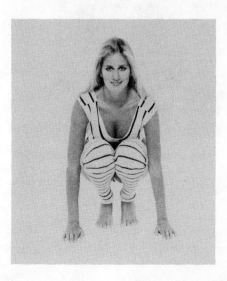

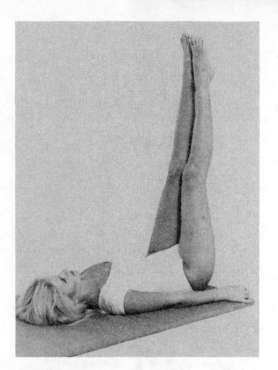

THE WALL WHACKER

Walk over to a wall and sit down in front of it. Now, lie down on your back and run your legs up the wall so that they are tall and straight and next to each other, and your buttocks are against the baseboard. Now, lean as far forward as you can, attempting to grab your ankle, pulling your head up to your knees. Hold your head there for ten seconds each time, and repeat five times on each leg.

Benefits: Excellent stretch for the back of the legs and for the lower back.

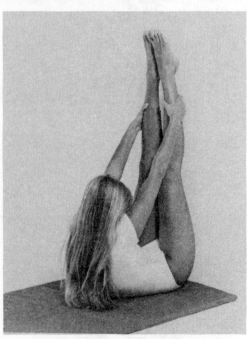

THE NOSE KNOWS

Begin by standing with your feet together. Now, take a step with the right foot, moving it about fifteen inches forward. Anchor it, and take a step backward some fifteen inches with the left foot, so that you have essentially done a small split. Grasp your hands behind your back and slowly bend forward, the bend coming at the base of the spine. Attempt to touch your nose to your right knee. As soon as you touch, bring your hands around and grasp your ankle, pressing your nose to your knee. Hold the position for fifteen seconds. Then return to the starting position, and do the same Sexercise with the left leg forward. Repeat each side five times.

Benefits: Stretches the back of the legs and knees, and adds flexibility to the back.

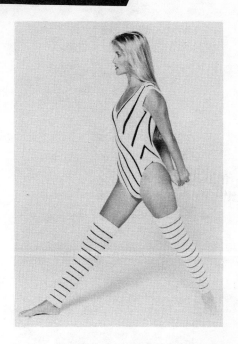

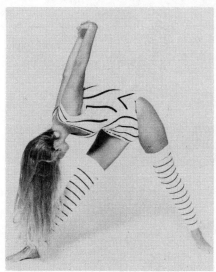

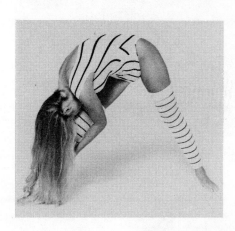

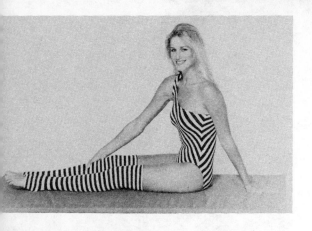

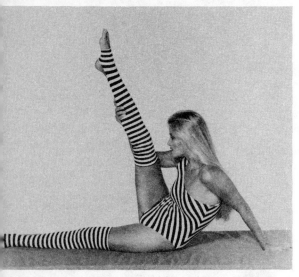

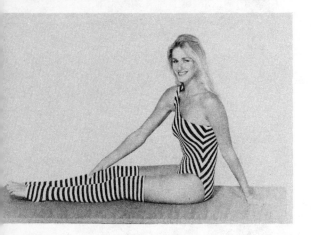

THE "N"

Sit down on the floor, legs extended in front of you. Grab your right leg at the calf with your right hand and bring the leg up toward you, while extending your left arm behind you for support. Lean back on your left arm, and bring your leg up to a vertical position. You should strive to keep the leg perfectly straight and vertical; the trunk can be reclining backward against the support of the left arm. Hold for five seconds, and then return the leg to its original position. Repeat ten times with the right leg, then switch to the left leg and repeat ten times. This is a perfect warmup for learning to do the Hoof-To-Mouth.

Benefits: Stretches and warms up the hamstring and calf, and adds flexibility to the pelvic region.

THE LAUNCH PAD

This one is terrific for building the legs and buttocks. Start by lying on your back, with your knees bent, arms down at your sides. The lower legs should be perpendicular to the floor. Now, lift your hips off the floor so that a line can be drawn from knee-cap to shoulders. Pretend that you are a rocket launching platform. There is an incredibly light rocket resting on you and you can aim it anywhere you want by pointing an extended toe. Bring your left leg up so it is perfectly straight, toes pointed, buttocks tight, and the line can now be drawn from toes to shoulder. Hold for a count of two; then, in a smooth motion, settle the hips down onto the floor, and as soon as they hit riase, them again. Repeat the movement ten times. Then, go to the neutral position, and do the same Sexercise using the right leg instead of the left. Feel the pull in the legs and buttocks. Terrific!

Benefits: Builds strength in legs and hips.

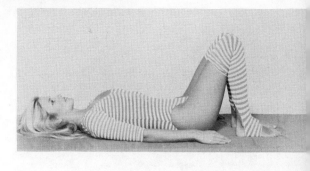

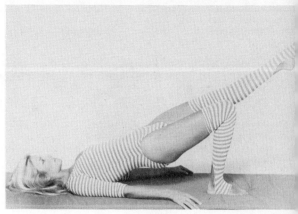

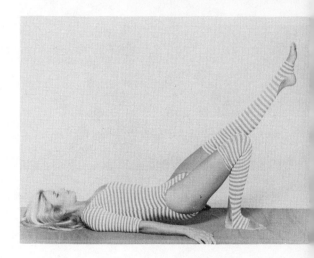

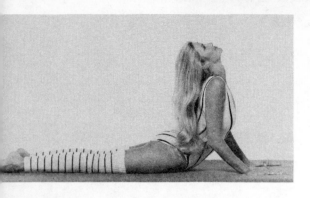

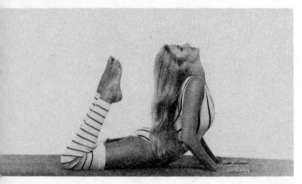

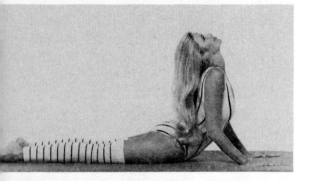

THE PRETZEL

Lie down with the front of your body on the floor. Now, stretch you arms out perpendicular to your body, using them as support. The object is to bring your legs together, and bend them at the knee, and get as close as you can to touching the back of your head with the soles of your feet. You will have to arch your back to make this work. Be careful that all movements are smooth and careful, and don't strain your back. When you arch to your maximum, hold for ten seconds, and then return to your starting position. Repeat The Pretzel five times.

Benefits: Offers tremendous stretch to the anterior part of your body and is good for adding strength and flexibility to the lower back.

THE DOG

Get down on your hands and knees. Now, keeping your right leg bent, and thinking of your right hip socket as a hinge, swing the right leg up until the entire leg (still bent at the knee) is completely parallel to the floor. Hold for a count of two, and then bring it back down. Repeat The Dog ten times, and then do it ten times on the other side. Nothing should move except the socket connecting the leg to the hip. As you progress, you can hold the leg up longer and longer on each swing. An alternative to doing ten times on one side and then ten on the other, is to do one on the right first, then do one on the left, and then two on the right and two on the left, until you total ten each.

Benefits: Builds strength in the sides of the buttocks and the sides of the thighs.

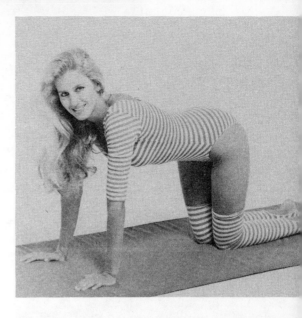

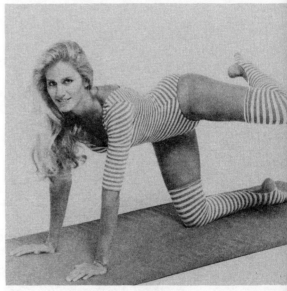

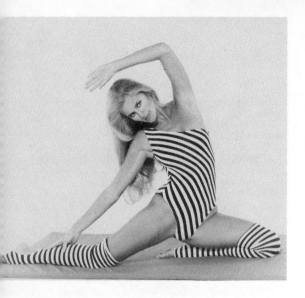

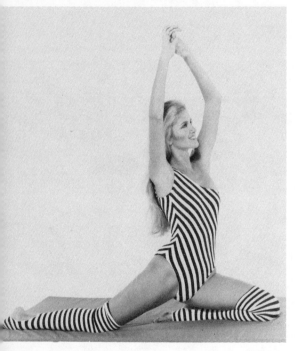

THE ARCH OF TRIUMPH

Kneel on the floor, and lower yourself back onto your heels. Now, shift your weight to your left leg and extend your right leg out behind you, making it straight. Your left toes grip the floor. Using your left leg as a sort of spring lever, raise your torso slightly and arch back so that you can bring your left arm up and over you, keeping it straight. Go back as far as you can; don't even hope that you'll be able to touch anything behind you with the left arm. Use it to stretch out the side. At the same time, slide your right hand along your right leg for support — and to extend your stretch even farther. Ultimately, your right hand should reach your right heel. After you have extended to your limits, slowly and gracefully bring your arms back up over your head, and when they end up in front of you, lower your head to your left knee, continuing to hold the arms out straight in front of you. Repeat The Arch of Triumph ten times to a side.

Benefits: Stretches the sides of the torso, adds flexibility to the waist and stretches the muscles along the front of the leg.

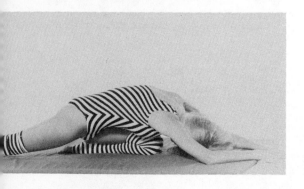

THE NET MENDER

This exercise has evolved from the style used by Filipino fishermen who squat in this manner when they mend their nets. From doing it daily, year after year, they have become expert at it. For those of us who do not daily mend our nets, it becomes something of a challenge. Stand on the outsides of your feet. Make sure that your feet are flat on the floor. Now, go into a squat and balance yourself by holding your arms out in front of you parallel to the floor. Hold the pose for thirty seconds, then resume standing, shake out each foot for about five seconds, and repeat the Sexercise five times.

Benefits: Terrific for stretching the Achilles tendon and does good things for the buttocks.

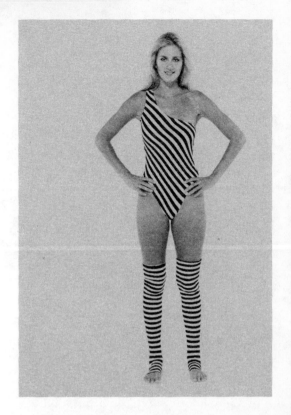

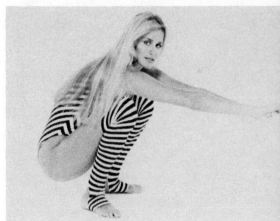

CHAPTER 3

Intimate Sexercises

If you have worked your way through the Casual Level Sexercises, you have two choices: stay there a while, getting more comfortable with them, or make your next quantum jump — up to Intimate Level Sexercise. The gap between Casual and Intimate is not wide. I intend to bring you along gently but surely.

On the other hand, if you are coming to these programs with considerable exercising experience, you may have skipped "Casual Sexercises," the previous chapter, and are ready to jump in right here. If you are an experienced exerciser, however, you know the importance of a good warmup and cooldown. The Casual Level Sexercises are more basic and easier Sexercises, which you might want to review for using as warmups or cooldowns. You could make some of them part of your regular exercise routine.

I hope that you are reading and using this book to improve your lovemaking. That's why I wrote it. I also hope that you are putting to good use what you've learned, and that you come to this chapter having done the exercises already described. And you should have attempted the accompanying lovemaking positions. Perhaps you've come across a lovemaking position that particularly fascinates, or that is new and interesting to you. Maybe you react as I do when I experience that unique position. I prefer to linger over that titillating pose, purposefully coming up just shy of perfection, so that I have to do more homework on it. If only school homework could have been so fun.

Before getting deeper into Sexercise, a few comments about the setting for lovemaking are in order. I think sex with the right person is good just about anywhere, any time. Traditionally, lovemaking has been associated with the bedroom. Realistically, that isn't historically true. If it were, none of us would be here, because our ancestors in the dim past obviously didn't have bedrooms in mortgaged houses. They indulged in sex right when the mood or the glands dictated — on a mountaintop one day, in the middle of a field the next. And people haven't really changed all that much over all those thousands of years. Some of you find sex excellent while camping in the Rocky Mountains, snug inside a down-filled sleeping bag. You are, of course, not limited to where you can have sex.

Some of the most memorable and exciting sex we can have is at the most unlikely places. I suppose that the threat of being caught in the act adds an alluring element of danger to the experience. But I've known people who've enjoyed sex in the back of a New York cab going down Fifth Avenue, in the middle of a golf course putting green and in the coach section of a jetliner making a transatlantic flight. Let's face it, you'd have a pretty short memory to forget an experience like that!

On the other hand, most people *always* have sex in a "standard" setting. They use the standard missionary position in the standard bedroom, using the standard bed, with the standard sheet ready to be pulled up over them after making love. You may think I'm going to be cynical about those standard-sex people, and make some wisecrack about how boring that is. But I'm not. One of the fascinating things about people is that there are so many variations among one species. There are some people who because of upbringing, society and their own inhibitions, would no longer enjoy sex one little bit if they deviated form what is standard or normal to them. And I'd much rather see them continue to enjoy sex to some extent, rather than have you or I harp on them to try it differently. It may get to the point that they feel pressured to try sex differently, but they are so up-tight doing it differently that they become self-conscious, guilty, bent out of shape, and they no longer enjoy sex at all.

Even the most libertine person on earth has certain limitations beyond which he or she will not venture. Everything is relative, which is much less profound than it sounds.

My point is this: even for the people who enjoy the standard missionary position, and who intend to enjoy that position with no variations, this book can be helpful. Doing the Sexercises in these chapters will build endurance, flexibility and strength, so that even the standard missionary position can be improved upon and more thoroughly enjoyed.

Some of you, even though you are liberal-minded and interested in expanding your sexual and physical horizons, will find that not all of the positions illustrated in "Casual Sexercises" are appealing. Some of them may be difficult, despite your being able to do the accompanying exercises and the exercises leading up to that difficult position. Maybe your body still hasn't adapted to the exercising program: twenty-five years of ignoring physical health is not totally reversed by three weeks of doing Sexercises. I'll admit, though, that there are a few Sexercises, even at the Casual Level, that I must still work on, not to mention some of the sexual positions. But it sure is fun working on them.

There are many reasons for having a hard time. It may stem from a childhood accident or the work you do; it may even be caused by wearing high-heel shoes. For example, a bad collarbone, resulting from a break, could affect your ability to do exercises employing the shoulders. Or, the typist who spends all day sitting at a desk typing, with his head turned to the right to read notes, could develop some muscular resistance to turning his head to the left, as might be called for in some of the exercises. Back to the high-heels. Wearing them too frequently can cause your Achilles tendons to shorten and lose flexibility. Then, when you exercise you may find that you have a restricted range of motion in the lower leg, ankles and feet. No matter what your limitation, do the exercises in this book regularly and, in time, you will see an improvement.

I had a surfing accident that damaged my ankle. I still find it very difficult to do exercises using that bad ankle, because it is so stiff. I routinely massage my ankle before starting my exercises. I also do some gentle movements to loosen the ankle. I find that helps. I must continue an exercise program for the rest of my life if I want to keep my ankle flexible and totally functional. The rest of my body will also appreciate the benefits of an exercising program.

But back to sex. Sex is like exercising, in that it can improve in leaps and bounds. Much of the improvement, of course, is because of attitude. Additionally, most of us go through phases with our sex lives. Sometimes we are consumed by it, while at other times it plays a surprisingly lesser role. And as we emerge from our time of sexual hiatus to take up a new relationship, we usually notice subtle changes in our techniques and our interests have taken place. In other words, our sexuality does not become locked into a pattern. As you change, so does your sexuality. Certainly, some people get into a rut with their sex lives and they seemingly stay there forever. Appearances, however, can be deceptive. A person might be experiencing major alterations in his view of sex; there may be a knockdown-dragout battle raging in the subconscious mind over this issue. The struggle is something of which he may have only a dim awareness. Some of these battles are lost and the person temporarily retreats from further sexual engagements. Some people also go through traumatic emotional and spiritual periods in their lives and totally withdraw from sex.

Getting into Sexercise can be the catalyst to another quantum jump in your sexual development. Do not look at your move from CasualLevel to Intimate-Level Sexercise as a jump of great proportions, however. Instead, look at it as a smooth transition from one level to the next. Changes in your sex techniques, caused by your ability to initiate different positions, will occur naturally, perhaps in the midst of a chapter. You should practice the exercises and the positions diligently, periodically reviewing them. As I've already stated, the homework can be quite enjoyable. Do not be intimated by moving into the Intimate Level. Just move into it smoothly and with confidence, doing the exercises and positions until you get them right, even if you must do them again, and again, and. . . .

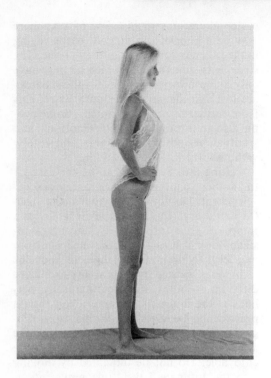

THE TUNNEL OF LOVE

Stand upright, straight and tall. Now, spread your legs out to your sides as far as they'll go, keeping them straight. Your legs should form a triangle, with the floor as one side of the triangle. Now, reach over, grasp your ankles and slowly and carefully pull yourself toward the floor, keeping your soles anchored to the floor. Go down far enough to touch your forehead to the floor and, using your head for support, rest in that position for thirty seconds. Then, just as slowly as you came down, pull yourself back up to a standing position. Repeat the Tunnel of Love five times.

Benefits: Stretches groin area, hips and back, while improving sense of balance. Builds strength in the back during the second half of the Sexercise.

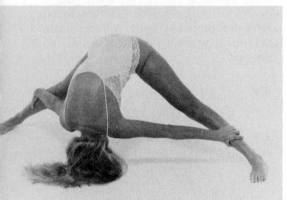

I SEE THE LIGHT

There is a theory that says everyone has an aura around his body. Some auras are supposedly stronger than others, and of different colors and hues. This Sexercise makes use of the theoretical aura. Begin by standing at attention. Spread your legs about eighteen inches apart. You'll start with your right hand, so put your left arm out of the way behind your back. Now, with your right arm, reach down to your right foot, following the progress of your hand, as though you were looking for your aura. Now, keeping your right arm as straight and stretched as you can, bring it up in an exaggerated manner until it is parallel with the floor. Pause for a moment; then, keeping your arm parallel to the floor, swing it behind you; keep it perfectly straight. Go as far as you can go, and then return it to the position out at your side. Continue on through that position so that your right arm is out in front of you, pointing straight ahead. When it is perfectly straight in front of you, pause a moment and then swing it back out to your side, still parallel to the floor. Now, swing it up above your head until it is pointing at the ceiling. Then, take all the life out of it and allow it to drop to your side. Repeat the same Sexercise with your left arm. Repeat ten times for each arm. You should be stretching during this exercise.

Benefits: Stretches arms and shoulders.

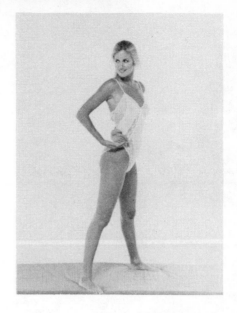

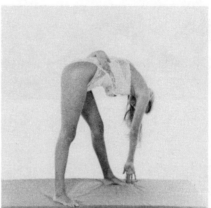

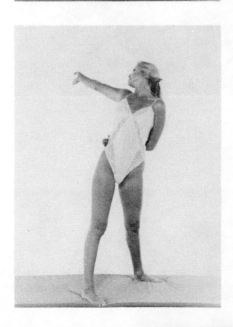

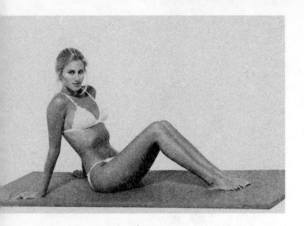

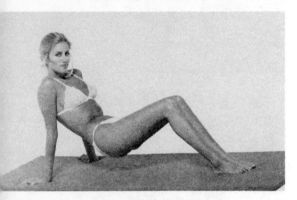

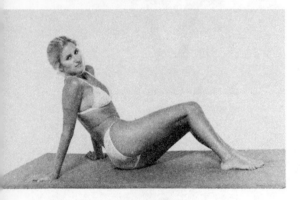

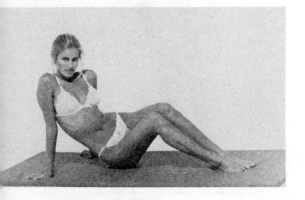

THE HIP TWIST

Sit on the floor, your legs straight in front of you. Move your arms behind you for support. Now, bend your legs slightly so that you can place the soles of your feet flat on the floor. Keep your stomach tight while you lift your hips off the floor. Twist your right hip down toward the floor; your left hip will face the ceiling. Gently touch your right hip to the floor. Return to the neutral position. Then twist your left hip downward, and drop it to the floor. Return to the neutral position. Repeat The Hip Twist ten times to each side.

Benefits: Builds strength in the arms, and adds flexibility to the hips.

PLAYING FOOTSIE

This one is excellent for loosening up the legs before or after lovemaking. It is also excellent before or after you run, cycle or ski. Sit on the floor, with your legs out straight in front of you, and your back straight. Bring your right foot to your navel. Do this by grasping your foot with your hands, and bringing it toward you slowly, bending your leg at the knee. The object is to touch your foot to your pelvic region. If you can't do it the first time, bring it as close to your pelvic region as you can — until you feel resistance in the leg. Then, return the leg to its starting position, and flex the other leg in the same manner. Do not be surprised if you find it easier to bring one of your legs closer to you. No one has equally flexible arms or legs. One leg is usually slightly shorter than the other, and the muscle development may be slightly different. Be gentle with the legs. Move them slowly. And when you meet resistance, stretch a bit right there, and then back off. Do this Sexercise ten times with each leg. Do not pull your leg beyond that point of resistance, or when you stand up you'll be walking sideways.

Benefits: Builds flexibility in the legs, and strength in the back.

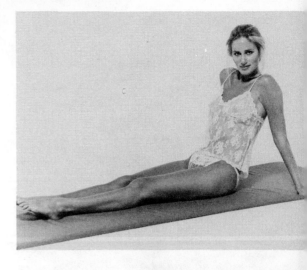

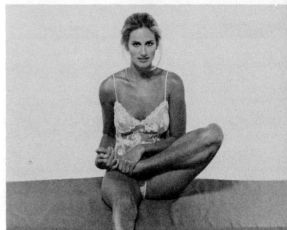

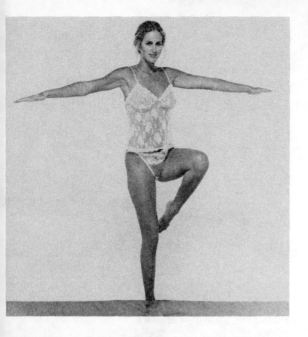

THE STORK

This is a Sexercise that develops stork strength. Begin by standing at attention. Then, lift one leg as though you were a stork lounging in the local pond. If you have to hold your hands out to the sides to maintain balance, that's okay. Hold the pose for one minute, return to your starting position, and then lift the other leg for one minute. Do this five times on each leg. Now, taking advantage of your warmed-up legs, lift one of them into the same pose. Using your arms to maintain your balance, bend the other leg and squat down. Once you are into the squat, hold it for five seconds, and then raise yourself back up. Return to your starting position, and squat with the other leg. Repeat The Stork five times to each leg.

Benefits: Builds strength in the legs and promotes a sense of balance.

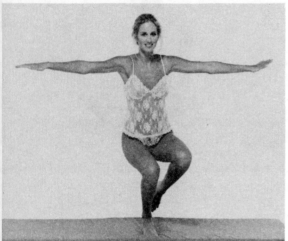

THE CRAWL

Here's one where you can swim without ever getting wet. Stand straight, and begin by spreading your legs about two feet apart. Now bend forward at the hips, keeping your back straight. Begin swimming motions, using the basic Australian crawl. Bring one arm up over your back, stretching it out far in front of you, dipping it into the imaginary water. Your other arm should be finishing the power stroke down through the water, ending up behind you, ready for the next stroke. Do this ten times to each arm; then turn your body slightly — to the right then to the left — and do ten more per arm, on both sides. Now wasn't that an easy way of getting in a swim without having to find a pool? As you become more comfortable doing this, you can increase the number of strokes, to as many as it takes to swim the English Channel.

Benefits: Builds strength in the arms and lower back.

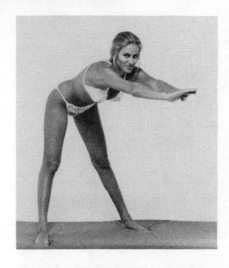

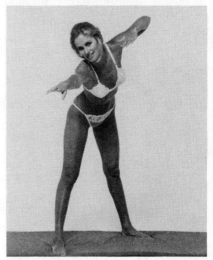

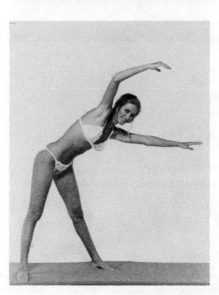

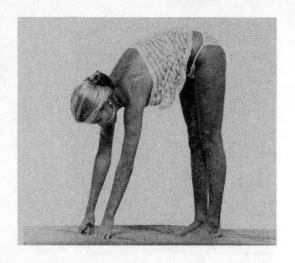

THE "Y" NOT

The object of this one is to look like the letter "Y" turned upside down. Begin by standing up straight. Then lean forward, bending at the waist, and place your palms on the floor in front of you, at a distance of about two feet from your feet. Now, raise one leg toward the ceiling. Get it as high as you can. Hold it up there for ten seconds, and then return; send the other one up now. Don't panic if you can't do this one at first. Like all exercising, you have to start somewhere. Repeat this Sexercise five times for each leg.

Benefits: Stretches the inner thigh and the backs of the legs.

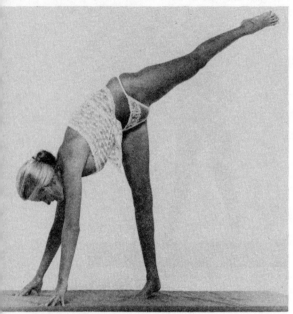

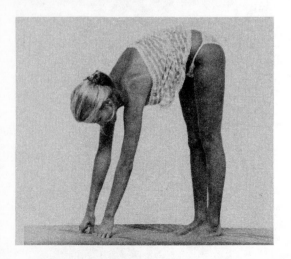

KNEE CLAPS

Lie down on your back. Bring your feet up toward your buttocks just far enough so that your lower legs are perpendicular to the floor. Now, using your shoulders to anchor your upper body, lift your buttocks off the floor, so that your body forms a straight line. Then, tightening your buttocks and maintaining that straight line, separate your knees about an inch and then bring them back together. Do it again, but separate them about two inches this time. Continue clapping your knees, each time increasing the separation between them by about one inch, until you can no longer hold yourself off the floor. Then begin clapping again, but this time *decrease* the distance between your knees an inch at a time. When your knees are finally back together, and the clapping is finished, lower your buttocks back to the floor. Rest for no longer than one minute, and then repeat Knee Claps one more time.

Benefits: Builds strength in the legs, the lower back and the buttocks.

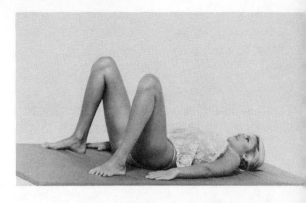

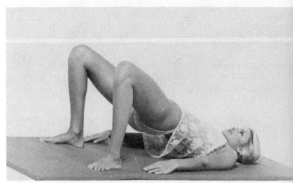

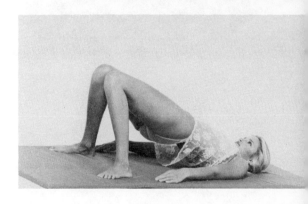

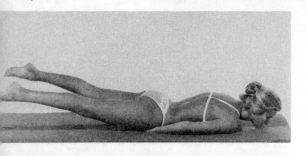

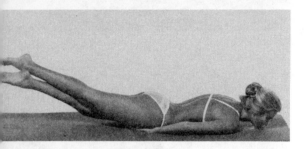

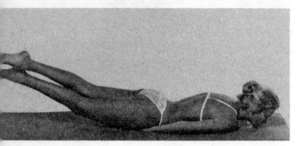

FRONT SILK CROSSOVER

This is essentially The Silk Crossover you were introduced to in the Casual Level section. The difference is that you'll be doing it upside down. In The Silk Crossover, you exercised while lying on your back. On the Front Silk Crossover, you should by lying on your stomach. Place your chin on the floor for support. Place your hands under your pelvic bones for support. Now, lift your legs up off the floor several inches. Spread them, and bring them back together. Send the right leg under the left, going as far as you can. Then spread them again, sending the left under the right. Do the Front Silk Crossover ten times, lower your legs and rest for a moment. Then repeat it ten more times.

Benefits: Builds strength in the legs, lower back and buttocks area.

THE INVERTED CRAB

Lie down on your back. Now, using only your hands and feet, pick your trunk up off the floor, very much like a crab or spider. Walk around the room in that position for thirty seconds. Lower yourself. Take 30 seconds of rest, and then do it again. Your arms should be cocked up over your head, and not merely pushed out behind your back. Once you get good at this, as you are walking about the room straighten out one leg and kick, pause, straighten out the other leg and kick, and then resume walking.

Benefits: Strengthens arms, shoulders and legs.

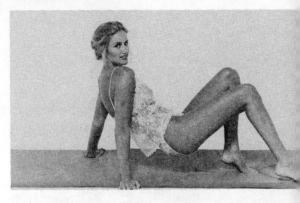

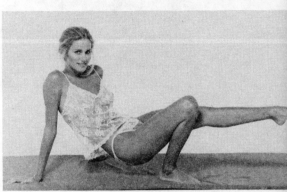

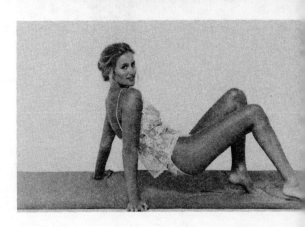

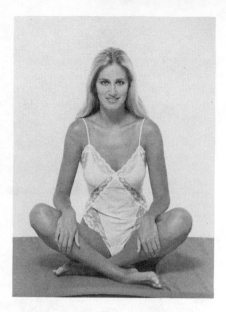

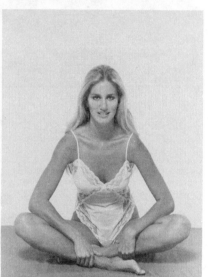

THE DELICATE BUTTERFLY

Most sex ultimately centers on the groin area. Yet the groin area is one of the most overlooked in exercise classes. Flexibility and strength in the groin area are extremely important for both men and women. This Sexercise is usually difficult for men to do, but once they've mastered it, they report benefits — in everything from more flexibility when playing sports to more fluidity in merely walking across a room. Start by sitting on the floor, back straight. Cross your ankles in front of you; if you are really agile, put your soles together; if necessary, you can use your hands to hold them together. Most men I know have a great deal of difficulty just getting into this position. If you are having problems, and can't get your soles together, don't ignore the Sexercise; bring your feet as close together as you can, and work from there. With your soles together, place your elbows on your legs, applying just a bit of pressure downward; when you meet the resistance, stop. Press very gently into the area of resistance, and then allow the legs to rebound. Now, flutter the legs up and down like a butterfly's wings for a count of twenty. Then repeat the slight pressure downward. Repeat the entire sequence ten times. The Delicate Butterfly is excellent to do while you're watching television.

Benefits: Adds tremendous flexibility to the groin area and to the inner thighs.

THE PETALS

If you can develop good flexibility in the groin area and along the inner thigh, you will have a great number of possibilities in sexual positions. The Petals will help in that direction. Lie on the floor, on your side, supporting your upper body with one arm. Now, raise your upper leg until it is perpendicular to the floor; hold it in that position with your free hand. Now comes the difficult part: Bring your lower leg up to meet the raised leg; do not help it with your free hand; it should continue to support the upper leg. Hold both legs toward the ceiling for a count of three, placing all of your weight on your hip. Slowly return the lower leg to the floor. Repeat this one twenty times, then roll gently to your opposite side and do twenty more off that side. Besides building a great deal of flexibility, this one also contributes to the development of hamstring strength.

Benefits: Builds groin flexibility and enhances hamstring strength.

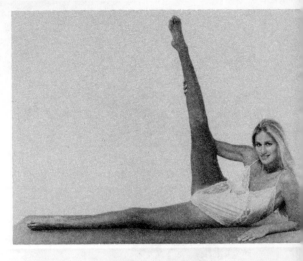

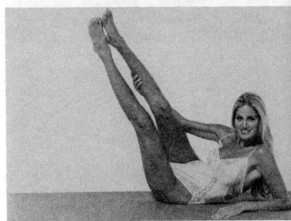

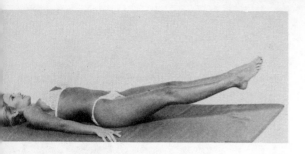

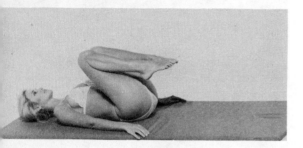

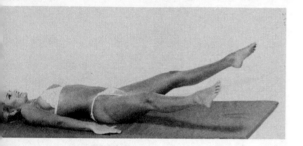

THE FROG LEGS

If you've ever watched a frog swim, you've probably been fascinated by the powerful stroke it makes with its legs. You can build that same type of strength in the legs by approximating the frog's motion. Lie on your back, arms at the sides, with the palms on the floor for support. Raise your legs four inches off the floor, keeping them together. Continuing to use your arms for support, bring your knees to your chest, keeping your legs together. The movement of the legs to the chest should be smooth but forceful. Be ready for the next movement as soon as your knees reach your chest. Now, quickly and forcibly kick your legs out straight, spreading them as far as they'll go. (Never do this one unless you are properly warmed up.) Immediately following the kick, bring your legs back together and, in one smooth motion, bring the legs back toward the chest. Repeat The Frog Legs twenty times, never touching your heels to the floor.

Benefits: Builds strength in the thighs, especially the inner thighs, and in the small of the back.

THE LONG REACH

For this one, start on your back, with your legs together. Place your hands on your hips and bring your legs up over your body, reaching your toes for the ceiling while keeping your legs straight. Use your hands to support your hips. Hold to a count of five. Now, still supporting yourself, bring the right leg down, bending it at the knee and running the foot along the still-straight left leg until it gets to the kneecap. Hold the position to a count of five. Now, making all moves slowly and deliberately, bring both legs down to the floor behind your head. This is a difficult position to hold, but try to maintain it to a count of five, making sure to hold the legs straight. Bring your legs back up to a reach-for-the-ceiling position, and repeat the exercise, using the other leg this time. Repeat the sequence five times with each leg.

Benefits: Terrific for the back muscles and for building up the backs of the legs.

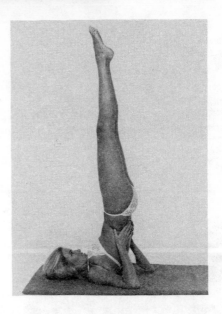

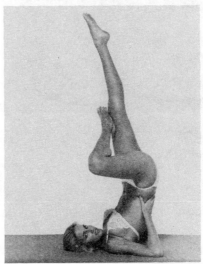

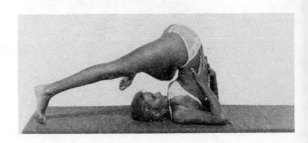

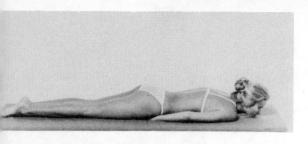

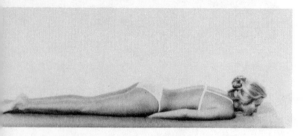

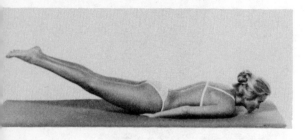

THE UPLIFT

This one is terrific for building buttocks and lower-back and leg strength. Start by lying face-down on the floor, your legs together, your face down, almost as though you were going to do a regulation push-up. You can place your hands under your pelvis. Now, plant your chin on the floor and in one smooth motion, keeping your legs straight and together, raise them as high as you can. The buttocks will tense up; you'll feel the strain in your lower back. Hold the position for a count of two, and then slowly lower the legs. Repeat this one ten times.

Benefits: Builds strength in the lower back and back of the legs.

SIDE SPLITTERS

This Sexercise combines strength and balance and works the inner-thigh region, the hips and the groin. Start by going into a squat, and then extend your right leg out to the side. Keep your hands just above your knees throughout the entire exercise. Now, keeping your back straight and trying to keep your head and shoulders from moving, bring your extended leg back in to a squat position. You should make all movements completely under control, and with as much smoothness as you can muster. Now, as soon as you are back into the squat position, smoothly move the left leg out to the side in an extension, again keeping the back straight. Hold for a second, and then return to the squat position. This Sexercise is essentially a half-split out to the side, and should be done ten times to a side. Side Splitters will help limber you up if you want to practice doing full splits; and if you can do full splits, you can let your imagination go wild on how you can incorporate them into your lovemaking.

Benefits: Builds balance, and strengthens the hips, groin and legs.

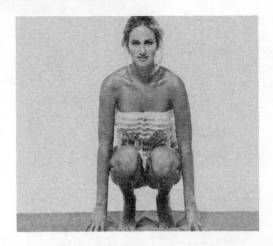

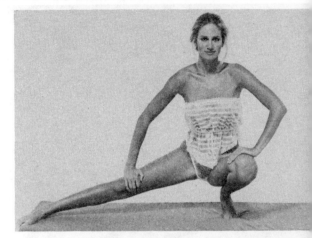

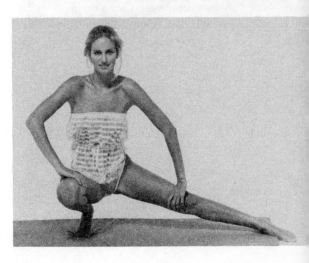

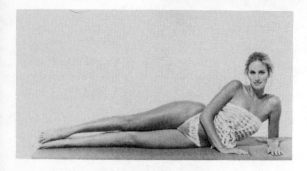

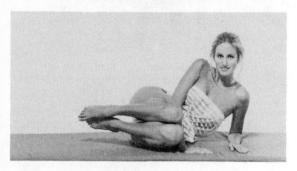

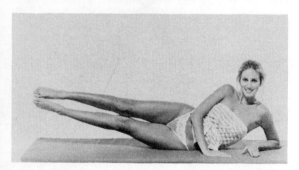

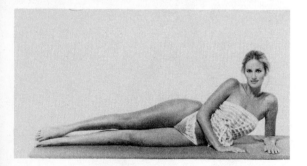

THE SIDEWINDER

This one may be difficult the first time through, because it requires balancing. But after a few tries, you'll be able to do it. Start by relaxing on your side for a moment. Now, raise your torso off the floor by using your elbow and hands for support. Keep your legs straight, making sure to use your hands and arms for support. Now, bring both legs up as high as you can, keeping them together. When you have your legs up as high as they'll comfortably go (until you either reach muscle resistance or run out of strength against gravity), hold them there for a count of five, making sure to keep them straight. As the count of five is completed, bring your knees forward, bending your legs, as though you were doing the sidestroke in the pool and you were going to kick away from the side of the pool. Hold them curled like that for a count of five, and then return them to the straight-legged position. Return your legs to the floor, rest five seconds, and repeat The Sidewinder ten times. Then, roll over and do it from the other side, with the opposite leg toward the ceiling. Repeat ten times on that side.

Benefits: Increases strength in the upper leg and lower back, while increasing flexibility in the pelvic region.

THE RAMP

This one looks, at first glance, to be extremely simple, and essentially it is. What complicates it is that so many muscles are used; it offers a good strength workout. Lie on your back, legs straight and hands at sides. Then, slowly and carefully begin to arch your back. Everything should stay on the floor except your pelvic region. The main contact points with the floor should be the heels of the feet and the shoulders. Hold your ramp for five seconds, and then slowly settle back to the floor. Take a deep breath, and repeat it four more times. This Sexercise is not indicated if you have lower-back problems.

Benefits: Strengthens back and adds flexibility to lower back.

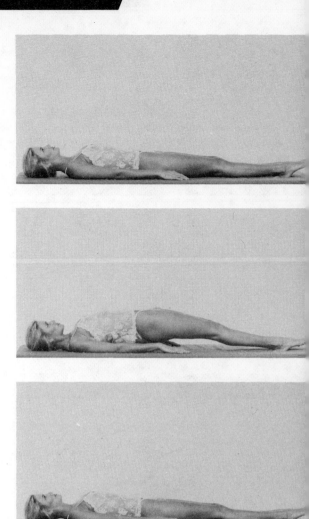

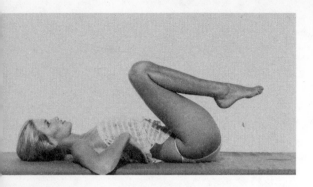

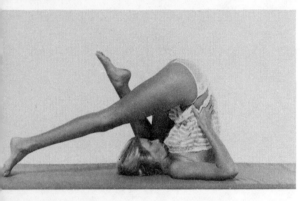

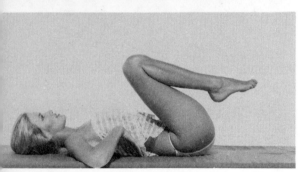

THE WEDGE LEG

This is one of the best Sexercises you can do for adding flexibility to your upper leg and groin area. You start this one by lying on your back on the floor. Grasp the sides of your chest with your hands, very lightly. You will form a triangle between the upper and lower arms and your sides, thereby creating a firm foundation. Now, with your legs together, roll them toward your chest, going into a tuck. Bring them over your head and, when you are balanced, reach them to the ceiling. Make sure that they are straight and together. Hold them there for a count of three, and then bring your right foot down your left leg. When your right foot reaches your left knee, stop. Keep your left leg straight. Now, tuck your right foot across the knee so that it is locked in place. Then, slowly and in complete control, roll your legs over your head, the object being to touch the toes of your left foot to the floor behind your head. When your toes touch the floor, hold there for a count of five. Your right leg should be in a very tight tuck under your outstretched left leg, and you should be feeling a pulling in the groin area and in the upper thigh. Don't push it beyond the point of stretching and into the region of pain. Now, slowly roll back up, aiming your extended leg at the ceiling. Slide your right foot up your left leg until they are together again. Hold to a count of three, and then reverse by bringing your left foot down your right leg. Repeat The Wedge Leg ten times to the side.

Benefits: Adds flexibility to the groin area and upper thigh.

THE LONG LEG

No, this one does not promise that you'll have longer legs after you've done it for three weeks, but it will stretch and strengthen your legs by some vigorous extensions. Start by supporting yourself on your arms. Now, bring your knees up to your chin. Then, begin extending your legs, in quick succession, kicking out forcibly, but very smoothly at the same time. You don't want to throw your hip out of joint, after all. But you do want the force of your kick to hyperextend your leg. This is very good work for the abdominals and certainly for the legs. Work very hard at making all your moves smooth and coordinated. Once your legs get moving, they should move as smoothly and as flawlessly as a bicycle racer pumping on level ground. Do The Long Leg twenty times on each leg, gaining speed as you become comfortable with it.

Benefits: Stretches and strengthens legs and adds flexibility to the hips.

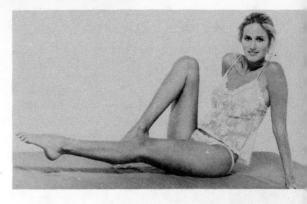

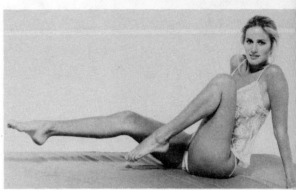

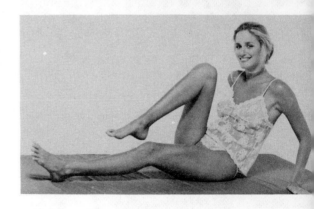

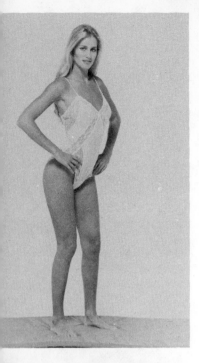

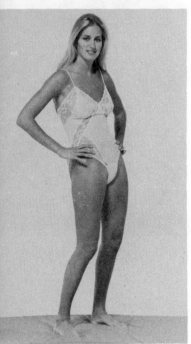

THE PELVIC THRUST

This Sexercise not only closely approximates a basic sexual movement — it is a sexual movement. But instead of doing it from the horizontal position, you'll be doing it form the vertical position. Stand up straight and tall, with your feet spread about eighteen inches apart. Now, place your hands on your hips. With a quick, smooth, powerful motion, thrust your entire pelvic region forward and upward, as high as it will go. If you've ever seen striptease artists, you have a pretty good idea of what to do on this one. It's the forward segment of the bump-and-grind. When you've thrust your pelvis out as far and high as it will go without throwing you off your feet, return quickly to the starting position and let your pelvic region relax completely. Then, without pausing, thrust again. Repeat The Pelvic Thrust I at least ten times.

Benefits: Strengthens the pelvic region and adds flexibility.

THE PELVIC THRUST II

This is pelvic thrusting in the horizontal position. You'll be in a standard push-up position, thrusting your pelvic region toward the floor. Start in the standard push-up position, and thrust the pelvis down and forward, shooting for the floor. On the return, allow it to bounce back up and then down to the neutral position. Keep the thrusts coming, until you've done at least ten of them. This is decidedly different from the Pelvic Push-ups, even though they are done from the same neutral position; in this one, you thrust the pelvis *down* and *forward,* and you are now swaying.

Benefits: Strengthens the pelvic region and lower back, and adds to flexibility of the hips.

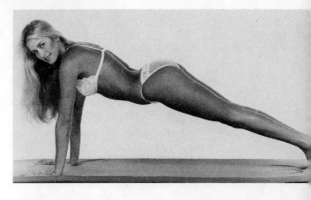

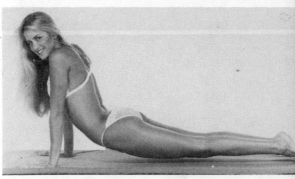

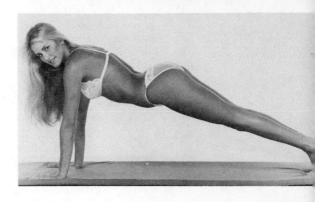

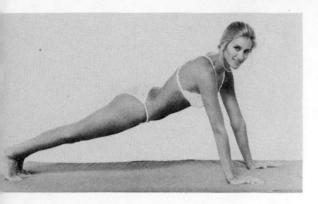

PELVIC PUSH-UPS

This is a rear-end variation of the basic push-up. Get into the standard push-up position, holding yourself off the floor on your arms (back and legs straight) and your toes. Instead of using your arms, however, you are going to keep them straight. Twist your hips slightly to the right; by that, I mean tuck the right side of your hip toward the floor, and then drop it that direction in a fluid and controlled motion. When it just brushes the floor, bring it back up to the original position; then tuck the left side of the hip and drop it toward the floor, returning as you brush the floor. Do this fifteen times to each side, and keep your movements fluid. All motion should be restricted to the hips and upper legs. Remember to keep everything straight, and use the hips.

Benefits: Strengthens the arms and shoulders, and adds tremendous flexibility to the hips.

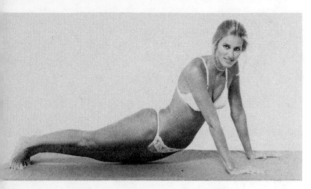

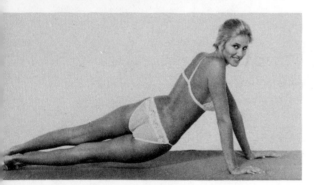

THE SWINGING BRIDGE

You can let your imagination go wild with the Swinging Bridge. Recall all of those jungle adventure movies where the hero has to cross a rickety swinging bridge to escape the crazed natives. Lie down on your back, and keep your arms to your sides. Bring your knees up, and plant the soles of your feet firmly on the floor. Now, raise your buttocks off the floor so that the points of contact are the soles of the feet and the shoulder blades. Now, swing your hips back and forth just like they are a swinging bridge and your hero is going to use them to escape. Do at least ten swings in each direction, then lower your hips to the floor, take a breath, and repeat the Sexercise again for ten swings.

Benefits: Strengthens the thighs and back, and adds flexibility to the pelvic region.

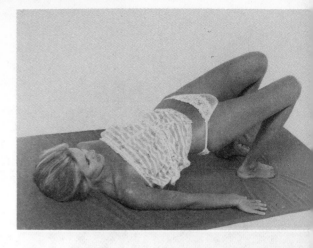

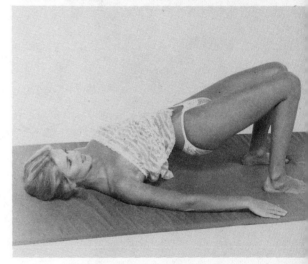

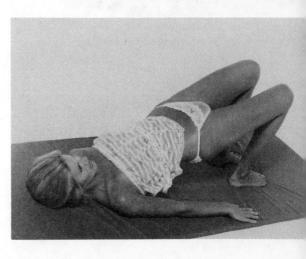

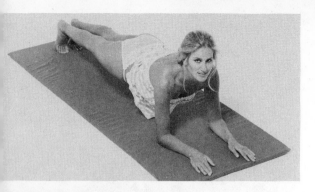

THE SWINGING BRIDGE II

This is a variation of The Swinging Bridge; here you will be doing the bridge by turning yourself over. Lie on your stomach on the floor. Now, bend your arms at the elbows, and place your forearms and hands on the floor for support. Then, lift your body off the floor so that the only contact points are your toes and your forearms. Begin your swinging motion back and forth, doing it ten times in each direction. Drop back to the floor for a rest, and then repeat it ten more times.

Benefits: Strengthens arms and shoulders, and adds flexibility to the pelvic area.

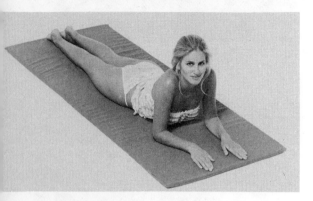

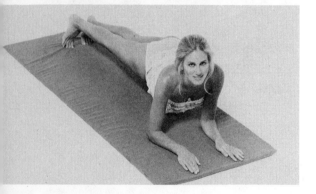

THE ABDOMINAL SUCK

Stand upright, heels touching, knees bent slightly. Place hands on upper thighs. Now, exhale as much air as possible out of your lungs. However, it is impossible to exhale all the air. When all the air is out, suck in the abdomen and attempt, by muscle control alone, to pull it upward into your chest. You should feel like you are breathing with the aid of the abdomen. Now, suck in air through the mouth and attempt to forcibly snap your abdomen back out by using the same muscles you used to pull it in. Pause a moment, and repeat the Sexercise. As you practice The Abdominal Suck, you should get to the point where you can do this ten times without a pause.

Benefits: Strengthens the abdominal muscles, and gives muscle control.

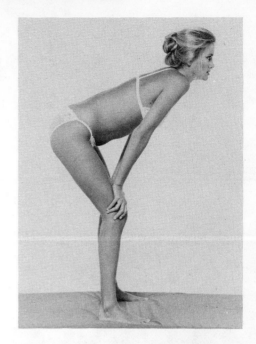

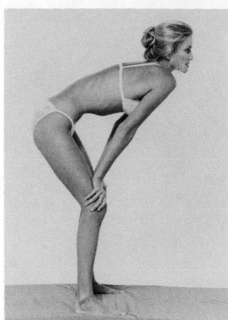

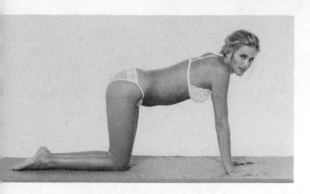

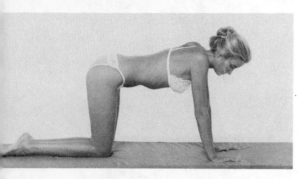

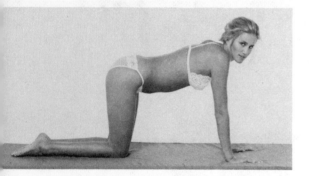

THE ABDOMINAL LIFT

Go down on all fours. Keep your knees together, and as you did in The Abdominal Suck, empty your lungs of as much air as you can. When you feel they are emptied, suck in your abdomen and hold it there for as long as you can. When you feel compelled to breathe in again, use your abdominal muscles to pop your abdomen back out. The object is to give your abdominal muscles a real workout by putting them through a very wide range of motion.

Benefits: Strengthens and firms the abdominal walls.

THE ABDOMINAL PUMP

Stand upright, heels touching, knees bent slightly. Place your hands on your upper thighs, resting them there firmly. Exhale deeply, emptying the lungs. Now, press down firmly on the thighs and pump the abdomen out. Hold for as long as you can, then breathe in and straighten to an upright position. Relax briefly. Repeat ten times.

Benefits: Strengthens and firms the abdominal walls, and builds strength in the upper legs.

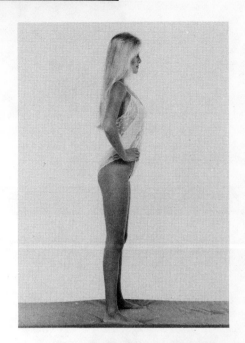

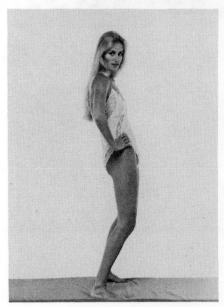

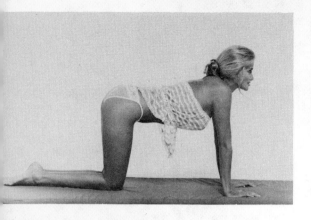

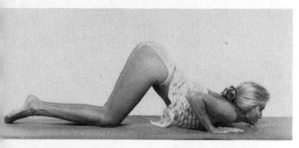

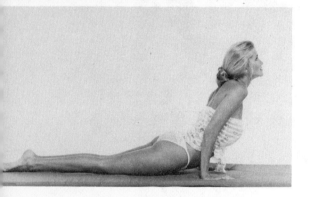

THE GROUND HAWK

This is a much simpler version of The Swooping Hawk from the Intense Level. Start on your hands and knees. The idea here is to imagine yourself as a hawk, personifying all of its graceful movements and fluidity. From your position on your hands and knees, go into a swoop by "diving" your head and chest toward the floor, allowing yourself to sink gently by controlling the rate of fall with your arms. Your back should arch because your hips should still be in the air. Now, as though you were a hawk attacking, skim the floor in front of you, and as you do, allow your hips to come down into the swoop. As you skim the floor in the front, push yourself upward, allowing your hips to follow so that you are back into your original position. It often helps getting started by backing up a bit; lean your entire trunk backward to give yourself a push toward the floor. You can do this by sticking your buttocks out behind you, and then starting the dive to the floor from that position. Once you begin The Ground Hawk, you should keep it continuous and fluid for about fifteen repetitions.

Benefits: Develops strength in the arms and shoulders, and stretches the back.

THE HALF UPLIFT

This one is done almost exactly the same as The Uplift, but instead of lifting both legs you lift only one at a time. Begin by lying down on your stomach. Place your chin on the floor and place your arms at your sides. Now, keeping your legs straight, lift one of them as high as you can, hold it there for five seconds, and then return it to the floor; immediately raise the opposite leg. Do The Half Uplift ten times for each leg. Don't be concerned if you can lift the leg only about two or three inches off the floor at first. Give it a chance. You'll be able to bring it up higher as you practice.

Benefits: Strengthens the legs, firms up the buttocks and builds strength in the lower back.

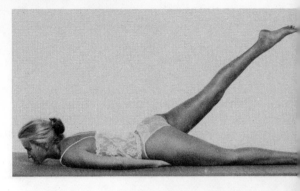

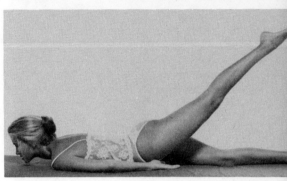

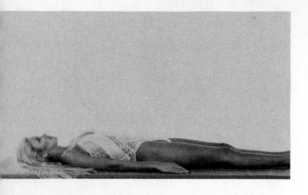

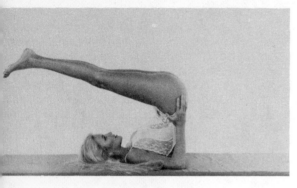

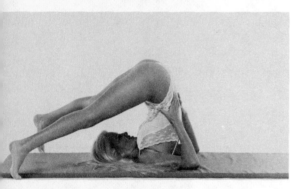

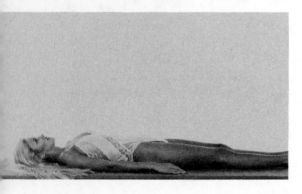

THE "V"

Lie down on your back. Extend your legs out straight. Now, place your hands under the small of your back for added support, and (keeping them together) bring the knees up toward your chin. Continue the roll until your legs are extended over your head, and keep them together. Now, supporting with your arms, grasp your hips with your palms to hold your buttocks up comfortably. Then, extend your legs toward the ceiling. Now, spread your legs, but keep them straight. Slowly, carefully, lower them over your head to touch the toes to the floor on either side of your head. Hold them there for a count of five. As you get better at this, you can bounce lightly off your toes as you gain equilibrium. But for the meantime, just work to touch your toes to the floor. If they don't touch at first, go down with them as far as they'll go; let gravity do most of the work. Do not overstretch and strain your back. Work on it faithfully and eventually you'll be able to get them down there with ease. Now, raise your legs back into a reach-for-the-ceiling position and pause for a second, before repeating the Sexercise ten times.

Benefits: Stretches the backs of the legs, the lower back, and builds the stomach muscles.

ROLL OVER, BEETHOVEN

This one is terrific fun. Sit down on the floor and cross your legs. Now, grab your left ankle with your left hand, and your right ankle with your right hand. Naturally, since you are sitting cross-legged, your arms will cross, too. Now, roll backward until you are on your back and shoulders, and as you reach that point, spread your legs wide, straightening them as you do so. Hold them there for about five seconds, and then bring them back in to a cross-legged position; as you do so, roll forward, ending up back in your sitting position. Repeat Roll Over, Beethoven ten times — or more, if you become fascinated by it.

Benefits: Stretches the legs and the groin area, and flexes the lower back.

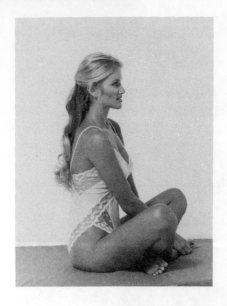

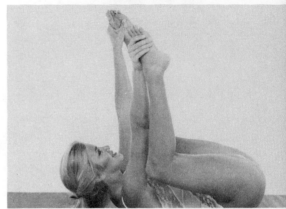

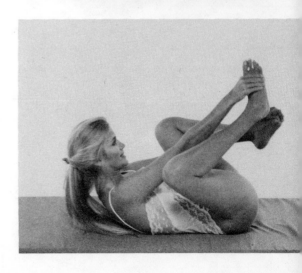

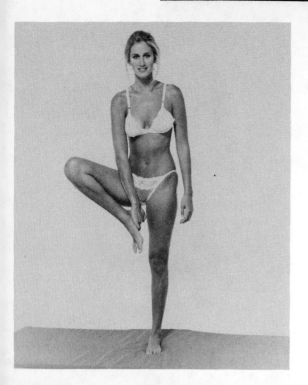

POINTER

This one requires a great deal of strength and certainly a good degree of balance. Stand straight and tall. Now, balancing on your left foot, bring your right leg up, sliding your foot along your left leg. When it is high enough to grab, take hold of the arch of your right foot with your right hand, and slowly bring the leg up so that it is parallel to the floor and straight out in front of you. There may be a tendency for your leg, because of your hip construction, to want to straighten out a little to the right side. That's okay, too. Don't force it straight ahead if it won't go that way. The object is to balance on your left leg, and to bring your right leg up and keep it straight. Hold it there for a count of five. Repeat the Pointer three times on each leg.

Benefits: Stretches the back of the legs, promotes balance and grace, and builds strength in back.

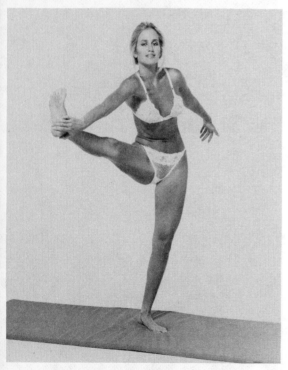

THE ULTRA POINTER

To do this you should have mastered the Pointer. Begin by warming up with the Pointer, doing three Pointers per leg. Then, go into the Pointer pose; but to further improve upon it, hold the pose and then slowly lean forward, touching your nose to your knee briefly, then return. This requires a great deal of practice, especially for balance. But the benefits are certainly worth it. Repeat the nose-to-knee three times on each leg, then go back into another sequence of three basic Pointers.

Benefits: Strengthens legs and back, promotes the sense of balance.

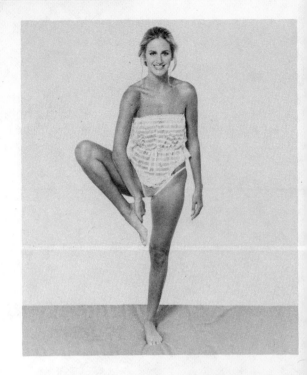

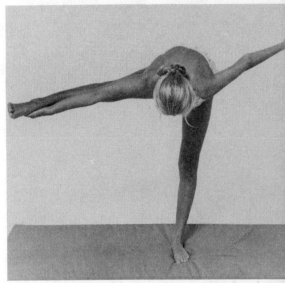

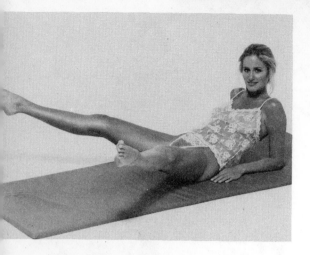

LEG SNAPS

Begin by lying on your back. Now, support your upper body on your elbows, so that you are comfortable and well-supported. Then, lift your legs about ten inches off the floor, spreading them apart as you lift. Now, bend the right leg and touch your toes to the left knee; then quickly snap your right leg back into a straight position, immediately bending your left leg to touch your toes to your right knee. Then snap it back to the straight position. This should be done very rapidly, yet carefully. It takes a bit of coordination, but it is exceptionally good for the legs. Repeat this twenty times to each leg. If you have had knee surgery or have knee problems, modify the snapping portion of the exercise so that it is not quite so violent.

Benefits: Strengthens abdominal muscles, stretches the groin area, and strengthens the legs.

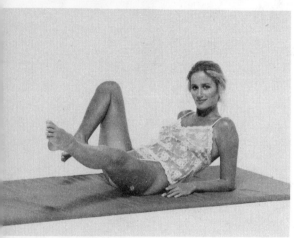

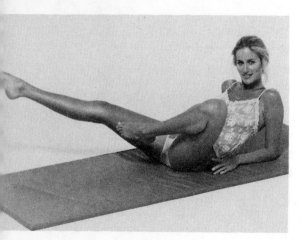

THE WOMEN'S PUSH-UPS

The standard push-up is not as simple as it may look. It requires a very straight back, and concentrates all of its benefits in the strengthening of the arms. At least for beginners, it is very much a male exercise, because men have stronger arm muscles. And, when you think about sex, the basic missionary position relies heavily upon the male knowing his push-ups. If you want to reverse positions and get on top, however, it is important to have strength in the arms. And a good way to begin adapting to push-ups is to do The Women's Push-ups, which are somewhat easier than the basic push-up, because you aren't required to push up quite as much weight. Kneel on the floor and, with back straight, hold yourself off the floor in front of you. Now, keeping the back straight and using only the arms, lower yourself to the floor. Take in a deep breath, and as you let it out through pursed lips, raise yourself back to the starting position. Repeat this one ten times if you can. Try to gradually work it up to twenty-five repetitions.

Benefits: Builds arm strength.

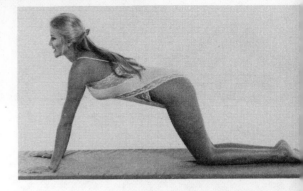

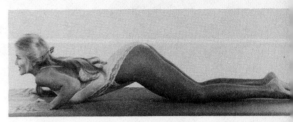

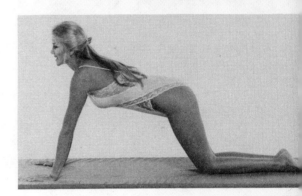

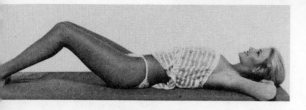

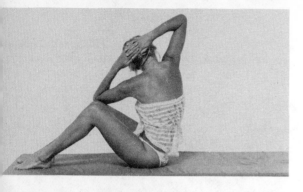

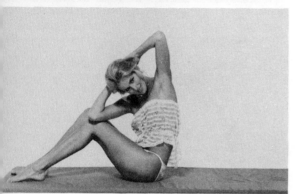

THE ALL-PRO SIT-UP

This sit-up routine is for the Sexerciser who has really got her program together, because it requires strong stomach muscles and good balance. Sit down in the middle of the floor, away from all furniture. Extend your legs out in front of you, and bend the knees just enough to allow you to rest your soles flat on the floor. Now, lie back on the floor, placing your hands behind your head. Normally, you'd anchor your feet to make things easier when you lifted to touch your elbows to your knees. This time, though, you're on your own. In a very careful, smooth, slow manner, raise yourself up onto your buttocks and keep going forward to touch your right elbow to your left knee. Return to the reclining position, and then raise yourself again to touch your left elbow to your right knee. This is going to be very difficult until you get it down because you will tend to lose your balance as you come up, your torso wanting to fall backward. Don't allow that to happen. That's why it's important to do this slowly. You should feel a strain in the stomach muscles, because this is where almost all the work is centered. If this is too difficult, you can bend your legs a bit more so that you won't have to bend so far forward when you come up. The ultimate object, though, is to have them as far down toward the floor as possible. Do this one ten times to the side.

Benefits: Does a terrific job building stomach muscles.

THE KNEES

This one may be a little difficult for you at first, as far as balance goes, but with a little practice you'll find it as easy as riding a bicycle. Drop down to one knee, keeping the thigh perpendicular to the floor. Now, plant the foot of the opposite leg flat on the floor in front of you, which means that your thigh is parallel to the floor, and your lower leg is perpendicular to the floor. The object of this Sexercise is to loosen and stretch the trailing leg (the one with the knee on the floor). Keeping yourself kneeling tall, reach behind yourself and grasp the ankle of your trailing leg with the corresponding hand, and slowly pull the ankle up until the heel of your foot contacts the buttock. Now, very slowly and carefully, lean forward on the leg you've pulled up. You should feel the stretch along the entire front of the upper leg. Lean into the stretch until it becomes just slightly uncomfortable, hold for three seconds, and then return to the original position. Repeat five times, and then alternate to the other leg. If you are having trouble balancing yourself on this one, it is all right to support yourself with your free hand, on a sofa or some other stable object.

Benefits: Stretches the thigh, and complements activities that work the upper leg and that tend to tighten it.

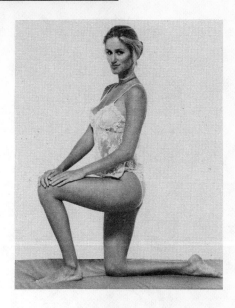

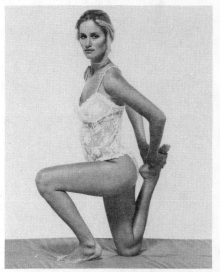

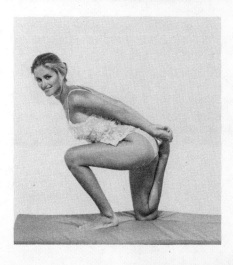

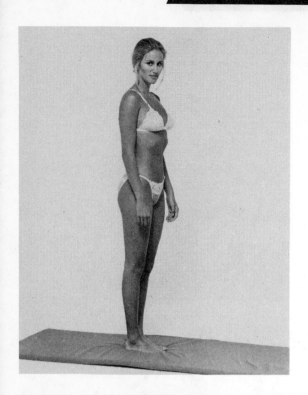

MILITARY DROPS

This one comes straight from the military, but it is a very effective combination of squats and push-ups. Begin by standing at attention. One the count of "One," drop to a squat, placing your hands on the floor beside your feet, palms down. Now, on the count of "Two," extend your legs out behind you, which effectively puts you into the standard push-up position. Now, do one push-up on the count of "Three," and then hop back into the squat position on the count of "Four," and on the count of "Five," resume standing. Now, put it all together and repeat Military Drops fifteen times.

Benefits: Builds strength in the arms and flexibility in the legs, and promotes good coordination.

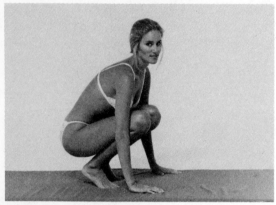

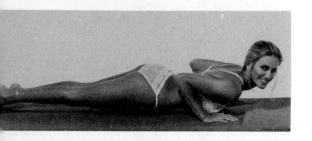

TIME

Imagine your body as the hands of a huge clock. Stand up straight with your legs two feet apart and put your arms down at your sides, and it's 6:30. Put your arms together over your head, and it's 6:00. Starting with that premise, you'll go through the hour between 6:00 and 7:00. Your legs should remain where they are. They are the small hand of the clock, and they stay at the 6. Your arms will form the large hand of the clock. Now, stand upright on your tiptoes, for a count of 1-2, 3-4, then, bending from the hips, stretch the arms out to the quarter-after-the-hour position for a count of 1-2, 3-4, then drop them to the thirty-minutes-after-the-hour position. Bounce lightly to an imagined beat, snapping your fingers or clapping your hands together to keep the beat. Now, springing from the legs, roll your arms up to the quarter-'til-the-hour position, bounce to the 1-2, 3-4 beat, and go back up onto the 6:00 position. Repeat 10 times, moving continuously through the face of the clock.

Benefits: Builds leg strength and flexibility, and stretches the arms.

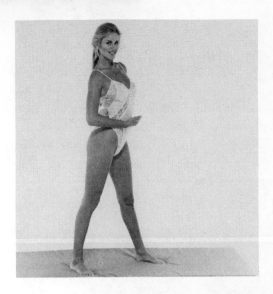

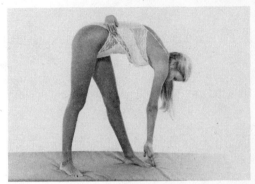

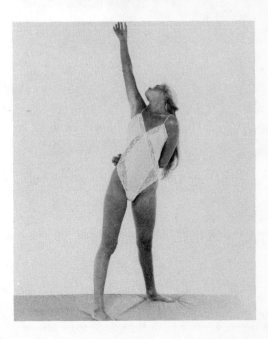

CHAPTER 4

Intense Sexercises

It is something of an understatement to say that the Intense Level Sexercises are not for everyone. The Sexercises contained in this chapter are designed to challenge your endurance, flexibility and strength.

Do not feel discouraged if these are too difficult for you to do immediately — or in fact, if they are too difficult for you to do ever. They are merely another level toward which you can strive in your continuing effort to reach your potential.

When I exercise after considerable traveling where I've had my regular exercising schedule interrupted, I find that I must ease back up to these exercises — very carefully.

If you have been carefully following the progression of the exercises through the previous two chapters and are just entering the land of the Intense, my advice is to tackle only one of the Intense Level Sexercises per session, adding one new one at a time. If any of them cause particular problems, merely pass over them, give them another try the next session and keep trying until they become manageable. Some of you might not have the right build to do some of these exercises, and if that's the case, don't feel guilty or incomplete because you are unable to do them. Sexercises such as the Spider Woman are particularly difficult, even for the experienced Sexerciser. Use common sense in approaching them — especially if you have had a bad back.

Remember, work these into your program one at a time. And do be careful.

I'm still bewildered by those normally sensible people who get into an exercise program and then abandon all common sense in an effort to reach the advanced level overnight. Believe me, it's a guaranteed way to get into and out of exercising in the same week.

The situation is a lot like that television documentary some years ago that stirred up so much controversy about Marin County, California. The program depicted that county as a place where the residents spend all of their time sitting in hot-tubs and stroking each other with peacock feathers. The program conveyed the notion that Marin County residents were "into" experiencing all there was to enjoy in the world; it saw them as being spoiled from having the income to literally buy anything they wanted. No more waiting for *anything*, the I-want-it-all-now syndrome. You want a BMW 320i?

Go get one. You want a house on a hill? No problem.

Let's face it, though. There are some people who are that way — people who get rich quick, people who go from paupers to philanthropists in no time. Those few, if they want it all now, have the means to get it. For most of us, however, there is a more "leisurely" route to getting everything we want.

As for exercise, some people have absolutely no patience with themselves. There are several things that can cause such a situation — and the problems that go along with it. For one, the exerciser may be so up-tight and impatient from her daily life that the mood carries over into exercising, despite the unique capacity of exercise to *relax*.

I've seen people rush into a gym looking as though they were trying to catch a train; they jump into their gym shorts and then rush through their exercise sequences as though they were facing a strict exercise time limit. After a few weeks you never see them again because the exercise didn't turn them into a new woman or man overnight. They feel exercising is a waste of time. You can't expect anything positive from that kind of an existence.

Then there are the competitive types, people who feel that they must be built exactly like the most finely proportioned person in the gym, overnight. They don't stop to think that the gym's Arnold Schwarzenegger has been working at it seven days a week for five years, devoting an hour or more a day to get fit and stay fit.

The competitive personalities also want to avoid the "easy" stuff. They want to go directly into the hardest exercises. They don't want to mess around with the kids' stuff. It's immediately go to the head of the class or forget the entire thing! People like this are asking for frustration or injury — or both.

You can't undo a decade of disuse with a week of strenuous exercising. We talked about the soft machine in chapter one and we used the Z28 for making an analogy to our bodies. Well, we can still use the car analogy when considering people who have allowed themselves to get out of shape. Consider a Model T that's been gathering rust in the junkyard for about thirty years. Then consider the antique-car collector who comes along to salvage it. He'll pore over it and consider it from all angles, and then he'll have it put onto a trailor and towed home, where he'll take it apart, piece by piece.

Worn parts will be replaced, but he may have to fabricate parts that are no longer available. He'll take the car apart down to the last bolt and then begin reconstructing it. It is a long, laborious process. But he does it slowly, carefully, lovingly.

People who get into exercise in order to refurbish their bodies should also handle themselves with such tender, loving care. They should not abuse themselves, in the first place, by letting themselves get out of shape, and then abuse themselves further by trying to get into shape faster than they can. It is a process that spells d-i-s-a-s-t-e-r.

Just because these are called Intense Level Sexercises does not mean that you should become *intense* about them. They are merely the next logical step in your program. If you can do some or all of them right now, that's just terrific. But that doesn't mean that they should be approached as a separate and distinct set of Sexercises. They should — in fact, they *must* — be integrated with the rest of the Sexercises from the previous two levels so that they are not too intense.

Many of you have probably learned to swim the hard way; someone throws you into a pool while yelling the admonition, "Sink or swim!" That's no way to learn how to swim, and the same goes for exercise. You don't just jump into it. The best thing to do with Sexercises — or with any exercises — is to ease into them. Look at Intense Level Sexercises as the climax to a good lovemaking session.

You didn't just jump right into a climax. If you did you must be pretty good at imagining climaxes. You start with foreplay, proceed to lovemaking, climax and then either continue climaxing or ease down afterward. (Imagine yourself being wired to a meter that reads your pulse during a lovemaking session. The line you would find on the graph paper afterward would look like the bell-shaped curve we have occasionally talked about. And that's how your Sexercise session should look, if it were to be graphed. Start slowly with Casual, work into some Intimate, then do some Intense when you've reached that level; now ease off by doing some Intimate and finish your routine with some Casual.)

Make the entire process an experience that your body can enjoy, and one that allows your body to adapt gradually. Don't abuse yourself during the exercise portion of your Sexercise lifestyle; save that for the sex phase of your Sexercising.

Be gentle with yourself, but work out frequently and well within your capacity. If you feel you can do more, increase the number of Sexercises. When the time comes to ease into the higher levels, do so gently and do only a few reps the first time, after you have built a good base.

It's your body, and it's the only one you've got, so take good care of it. Make it sleek and ready for action, and then use it as often as you want. Half the fun, as with foreplay, is getting there. You know what I mean?

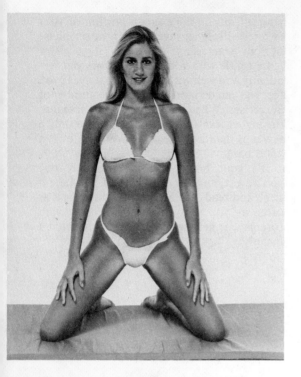

THE MOLE

This one is fun and stretches many of your muscles as well as it stretches the imagination. The part that makes it an Intense Level Sexercise will quickly be noticed. Start by kneeling on the floor. Give yourself plenty of open floor space in front of you. Now, spread your knees about two feet, so that a "tunnel" opens between your legs. Now, the object is to pretend you're a mole and to burrow down between your legs. Put your hands and arms in there first, and then your head, tucking as much of yourself in there as you can manage before your position and the curve of your back cause you to roll forward. The object is to get in as far as possible before you roll. The better you get, the farther you'll be able to crawl into yourself before you begin to roll. Repeat The Mole ten times. There is a variation of this one that marks a real expert. Following the inevitable roll, try to reverse the entire process. I know, it isn't easy. But once you get flexible enough, it *is* possible.

Benefits: Builds tremendous flexibility in the back and shoulders.

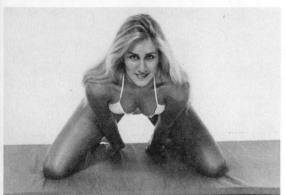

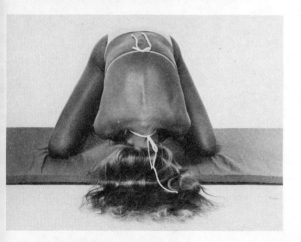

THE PENDULUM

Using a counter top or a chair arm that comes up to hip-level, stand about 2½ feet away from it, with your right side facing it. Now, raise your right leg and place your right heel on the counter top or chair arm, keeping your leg straight. Ideally, the counter top or chair arm should be at the same height as your hip, so that when your heel is resting on it, your right leg is parallel to the floor. Now, keeping your left leg straight, bend forward at the waist, keeping your upper body straight and your arms extended up over your head as though you were diving into a pool. Now, touch your joined fingers to your left toes, hold for a count of five, and return to your upright position. Repeat ten times. Then return to your starting position, and turn yourself so that you can raise your left leg and repeat the Sexercise ten times on that side. Return to the starting position, do a dozen toe-touches, and repeat the entire Sexercise, again doing ten reps to the side.

Benefits: Builds strength in the legs and flexibility in the waist.

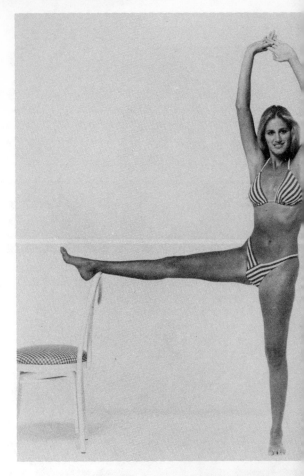

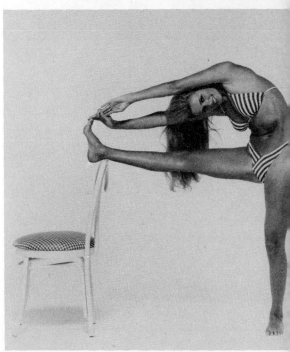

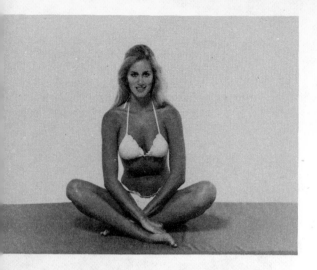

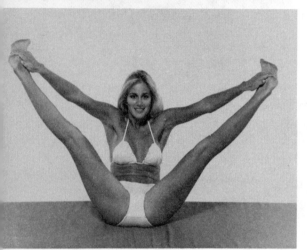

THE BLOOM

This one is referred to as The Bloom because it approximates the blooming of a flower. It requires balance and flexibility and is excellent for developing the legs. Sit on the floor cross-legged, back straight. Grasp your right heel in your right hand, and left heel in the left hand. Now, concentrate on making your movements smooth and flawless. Balancing yourself on your buttocks, bring your legs out straight. They should be at between 45- and 90-degree angles, depending on your flexibility. If you can't get the legs straight at first, do as best you can. Repeat this one five times, holding for at least five seconds once the bloom has fully opened.

Benefits: Develops strength in the legs, general body balance and flexibility in the pelvis.

FROGLEG BACKSTROKE

Begin by sitting on the floor. Extend your arms out behind you to offer support for your trunk. Then, raise your legs out in front of you at a 45-degree angle from the floor, keeping them straight and together, balancing on your buttocks. Concentrate on holding everything in place for five seconds. Now, keeping the arms and body perfectly still and in place, and concentrating all movements in the legs, bring them toward you as you bend them, spreading them in the process. Bring only your feet together, touching your feet to your buttocks. Do it all in one quick, smooth, powerful motion, the same way a frog kicks off from a lily pad. As soon as your feet touch your buttocks, thrust your legs back into the air into their original position. This Sexercise is excellent for strengthening your abdominal muscles and for adding a degree of flexibility to the groin area and the legs. Repeat Frogleg Backstroke ten times, making sure that you keep all movements smooth and controlled. You should not explode into the kick in such a way that you'll injure your legs. Control the action with your muscles to restrain the legs from kicking too far.

Benefits: Strengthens the abdominals and adds flexibility to the groin area and the legs.

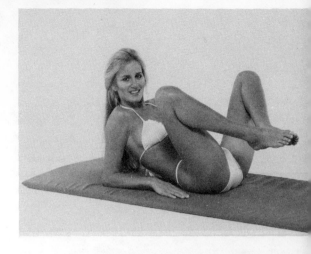

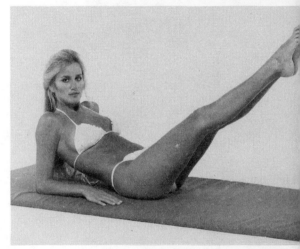

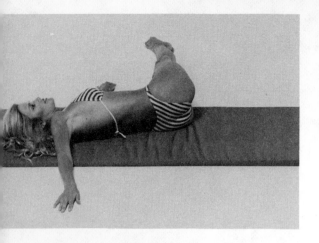

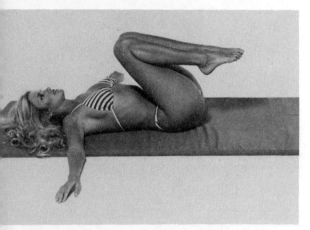

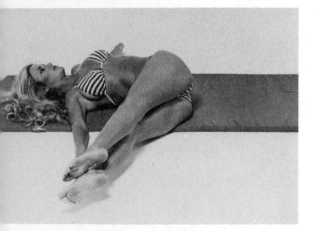

THE ROLLER

This one really puts your legs, hips and abdominals to work. Start out on your back, with your legs together and pulled up to your chest. Extend your arms out at 90 degrees from your body to supply a wide area of support. Roll your legs to the right, keeping them tucked and together. When your legs are on the right, about four inches off the floor, stop; extend your legs until they are straight, still keeping them together, so that the feet are about four to six inches off the floor. Keep the head, back and arms stationary, and make all movements from the hips. Now, with the legs extended, bring them around in a large circle, keeping them extended and just off the floor. When they reach a point on your left side equal to shoulder-level, bring them toward you in a tuck, and when they are back in (still four inches off the floor), roll at the hip until they are out to the right side, doing the entire movement again. Repeat this ten times, and then reverse direction for ten more.

Benefits: Terrific Sexercise for building strength in the abdominals and thighs, and for building flexibility in the pelvic area.

SPLIT FORWARD

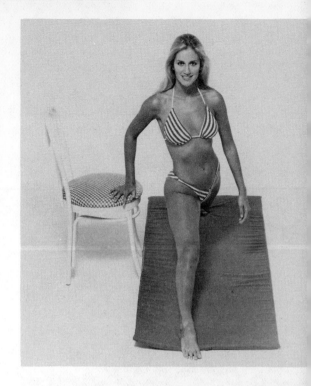

The split we all commonly imagine, especially when thinking of acrobats, circus performers or ballet, is the forward split: The performer sends one leg forward and the other back and slowly sinks to the floor until both legs are horizontal to the floor. I don't expect you to be able to perform a split flawlessly at first. To start, you can do a split by pulling two kitchen chairs out, setting them facing each other in the center of your exercise area, and then standing between them. Now, go into a crouch and place the palm of one hand on each chair. Stretch your right leg out straight in front of you, and slide the left leg out behind you. Now, very slowly, lower yourself into a split position. Don't expect to get all the way down the first time. Remember to keep your legs perfectly straight, and use your arms to control the rate of descent. Being very careful, lower yourself as far as you can *comfortably* go. Your legs will feel tight as you reach your comfortable limits. Lower yourself just into the area of tightness, hold yourself there for a count of five, and then bring yourself back up to the crouch; reverse legs, and start again. Repeat the Sexercise five times to each side. Eventually, and by working at it faithfully, you should be able to begin doing this without the chair.

Benefits: Strengthens the arms, stretches the fronts and backs of the upper legs, and stretches the groin muscles.

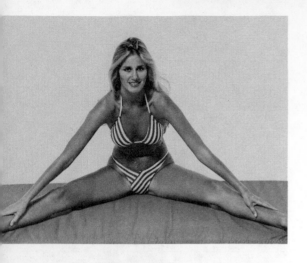

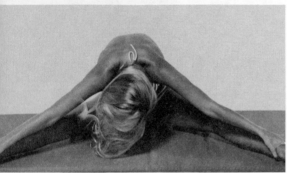

SPLIT SIDEWAYS

The second type of split is one that gymnasts do frequently. Sit down on the floor, with your legs out straight in front of you, and then bring your legs out to your sides, so that ultimately, you could draw a straight line between the big toes of your feet. Place your palms on the floor in front of your groin for support. This Sexercise requires a great deal of work, especially at the basic level of stretching and loosening the groin area. Many of the Casual Level Sexercises are specifically designed to work toward allowing you to more comfortably do this Sexercise; do not jump right into this and hope to do it flawlessly the first time, unless you are extremely flexible. Instead, work up to it. Sit down on the floor, your legs out straight in front of you. Place your palms on the floor behind your buttocks for support. Now, slowly begin to spread your legs, keeping both legs straight. Spread them until you meet resistance and then go about a half-inch into the resistance and hold for a count of five. Return the legs to the starting position and pause for a count of five, and then repeat the Sexercise five times. As you get to the point where your legs reach a straight line from toe to toe, begin sitting up straight instead of supporting yourself from behind. Be patient; take your time and work on it over a period of months. As you become more proficient, add the variation of sliding your hands down your legs to your ankles, and bobbing your forehead toward the floor in front of you; repeat 10 times.

Benefits: Stretches and strengthens the legs, and stretches the groin muscles.

SPLIT SIDEWAYS SUPREME

Once you have conquered the Split Sideways, you can take it one step farther and build additional strength and flexibility in your arms, groin and legs by adding this simple step. Once you have reached the optimum stretch, with both legs extended to the sides and your palms planted on the floor in front of your groin for support, get your upper body weight over your arms and push yourself up so that all that's touching the floor is your palms and the insides of your feet. Now, slowly bring your body weight all the way over your arms, so that if someone were looking at you from the back, your legs would be forming an A-frame. Hold for a count of five, and then slowly — and under complete control — return to your original position. Repeat this one five times. As you get this one down, add the variation of stretching out over one extended leg, returning to an upright position, and then stretching out over the other extended leg, once again returning to the neutral position. Repeat this variation five times to the side.

Benefits: Builds arm strength; stretches legs and groin muscles.

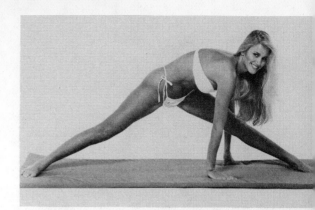

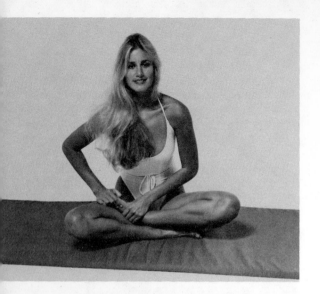

THE TIPPING LOTUS

Sit on the floor, legs out straight in front of you. Now, bend one leg at the knee and bring the ankle onto the opposite thigh. You can use your hands to put everything in its proper position. Now, bend the straight leg and bring it over the one that's already bent, settling it down on top of the other thigh; go into the basic lotus position used in yoga. Keep your back straight. Hold this position for five seconds, resting your hands on your knees. Now, bend forward at the waist, touching your head to the floor in front of you. Hold your forehead to the floor for a count of fifteen, then return to the sitting position. Repeat five times. This one will put strain on the knees and will also put strain on the lower back, so do it carefully and slowly, and if you are not able to go all the way through the Sexercise at first, merely go to the point of resistance and hold there. Eventually you'll be able to go through the entire range of motion — if you keep working at it.

Benefits: Stretches the inner thigh and the back, while also working on the knees.

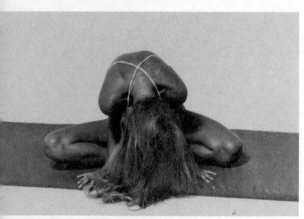

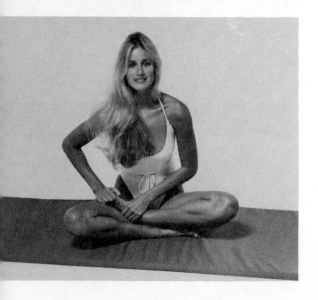

HEEL PLAY

Begin this one by lying on your back. Stretch your arms out perpendicular to your body. And spread your legs apart about three feet. You now have four potential contact points with the floor: your hands and your heels. Now, using those contact points, lift your trunk and legs off the floor. Ironically, the less you lift them off the floor the better. In other words, it is more difficult for you to hold the position with your body one inch off the floor than it is ten inches off the floor. Hold it at the point where it is most comfortable to start. You can always improve in this one and hold yourself a mere inch off the floor once you get really good at it. Hold for a count of ten, lower yourself back onto the floor, and repeat this one five times.

Benefits: Builds arms and leg strength, and stretches entire front of body.

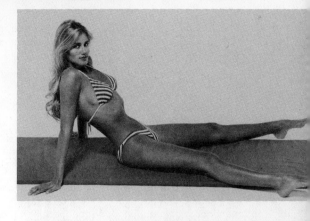

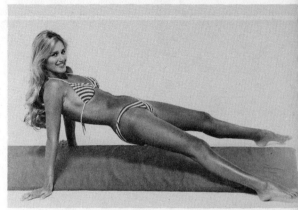

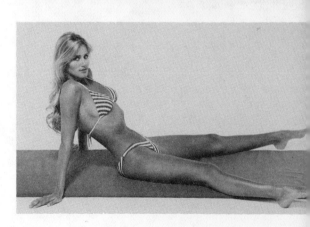

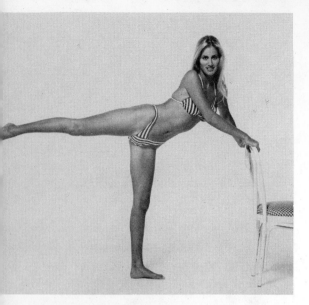

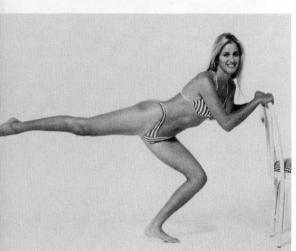

COUNTER SQUAT

Stand facing a counter or a table. Place your palms on the edge of the counter or table, and then back up just enough to stretch your arms out straight. Now, extend your right leg out behind you, keeping it straight. Then, begin doing deep-knee bends using only your left leg, keeping everything else immobile, and supporting yourself by keeping your hands on the counter. Do twenty on the left leg, and then change to the right leg, doing twenty more. Now, change back to the left and do ten more, then back to the right, and do ten more there. Finish by putting both feet back on the floor, and do ten regulation deep-knee bends. This should not be done, of course, if you currently have knee problems or if you are prone to them.

Benefits: Builds strength in the legs.

THE BUST BRIDGE

This one takes a good deal of dexterity, and certainly improves flexibility in the lower back. Start by kneeling on the floor, and lower your thighs onto your lower legs and feet. Keep your back perfectly straight, and lightly touch the floor with your finger-tips. Now, in a slow, smooth motion, lean your body backward, helping yourself down with your hands. Lower yourself very, very slowly. Of course, if you are prone to back problems, The Bust Bridge should not be done until your back muscles are strengthened. Continue to lower yourself until you meet the floor with the back of your head, and then allow your back to rest on the floor. Hold for one minute. Now, if your back is strong enough, slowly raise yourself into the upright position without the aid of hands and arms. If you are not quite strong enough for that, you are certainly allowed to use your hands and arms until you can do it without them. Do this one a total of five times, but keep it slow.

Benefits: Great for strengthening and adding flexibility to the back; also strengthens the thighs.

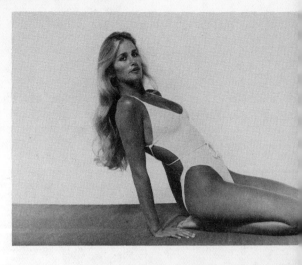

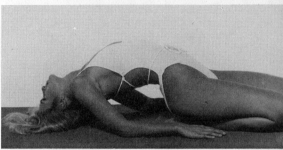

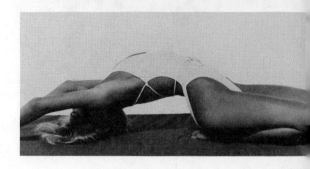

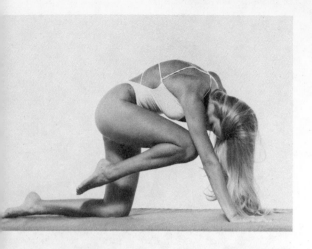

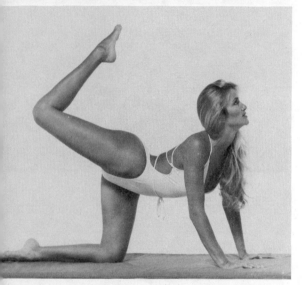

THE KWICK KICK

This one is terrific for stretching the legs, hips and the entire frontal area, and offers great inroads to flexibility. Kneel on the floor, head up and back straight. Try to make all moves coordinated and fluid, and keep them completely under control. This caution is especially important when going into the first movement. Bring your right leg up under yourself; while dipping your head, attempt to *lightly* touch your chin to your knee. While making the movement, round the back. As you can see, a miscue could be dangerous. Now, with a smooth motion, simultaneously shoot your legs back behind you and aim it for the ceiling, arch your back, and bring your head up. Keep your mouth closed to further exaggerate the beneficial stretching to the front of the body. Repeat this sequence ten times, and then switch over to the opposite leg and repeat the exercise on that side.

Benefits: Stretches entire front of the body and builds leg muscles.

CEILING TOUCH

Lie on your back, legs straight and together, arms immobile at your sides. Now, if you've ever seen any of the Esther Williams films, you've seen the syncopated swimmers floating on their backs, then raising their legs up toward the sky, keeping them straight, and slowly bringing them into the water. Do the same thing, but you needn't worry about sinking. Slowly and carefully raise your right leg up toward the ceiling, keeping it straight all the time. Now, when it is perfectly perpendicular to the floor, and without using your arms, raise your hips toward the ceiling, thereby pushing the leg even closer to the ceiling. All movement should come from the hips, with your points of contact with the floor being your left heel, your shoulders and your arms lying immobile on the floor. Hold for five seconds, and then lower yourself. Repeat ten times. Alternate legs.

Benefits: Strengthens the back and legs, and adds mobility to the hips.

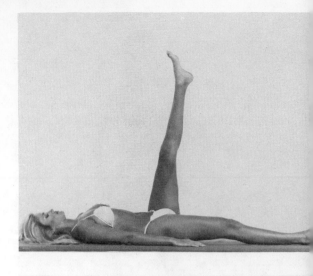

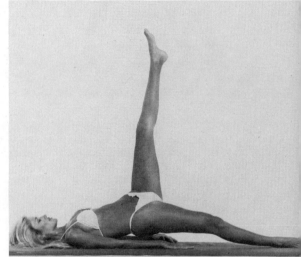

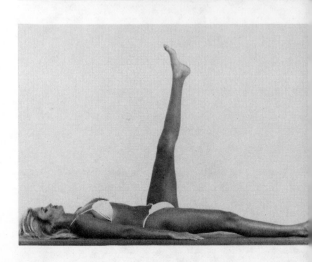

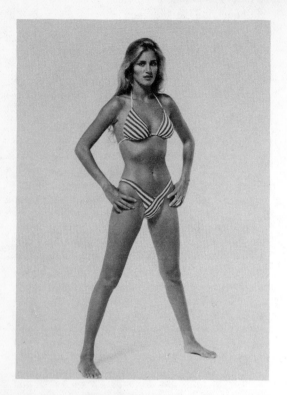

SPIDER PUSH-UP

This one is very similar to the standard push-up, and it will also be similar to one position of The Swooping Hawk, but is a Sexercise all its own. Begin by standing up straight, with your legs about two feet apart. Now, bending at the hips, drop to the floor so that your hands are planted, palms down, on the floor in front of you, and your buns are sticking up in the air. What you should have, then, are your palms and your toes on the floor, and your rump reaching toward the ceiling. You should look similar to a pyramid, or to a four-legged spider. Now, do a push-up, touching your nose to the floor in front of you, using only your arms, lowering your body only on the pivot of your toes. Pretty difficult, huh? Do ten of them. And, once you get that down, you can make it a little more difficult by raising yourself up onto your fingertips and doing it that way.

Benefits: Builds arm strength, while also building strength in the back and the legs.

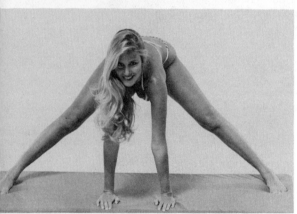

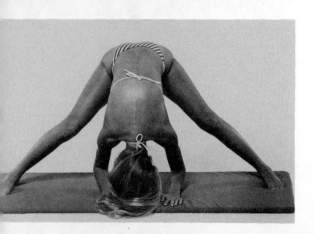

THE SWITCHBLADE

All Intense Level Sexercises should be eased into; push yourself only as far as your body will allow you to go, until it learns to move a bit farther with each try. Everything with Sexercises is a matter of gradual adaptation. For The Switchblade, lie on your back and place your arms at your side for support. Keep your legs together and straight, and carefully bring them up. Bring them over yourself, aiming your pointed toes at the floor behind your head. When the toes finally make contact with the floor behind your head, stop there. Now, with the toes on the floor behind your head, spread your legs at the knees just enough so that they can come up around your head, and bring them to rest on the floor, next to your ears. Bob up and down about two inches very gently, flexing your buttocks while doing so. Slowly and carefully return to the starting position and repeat the Sexercise five times.

Benefits: Strengthens the back and adds flexibility to the back and legs.

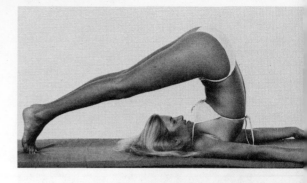

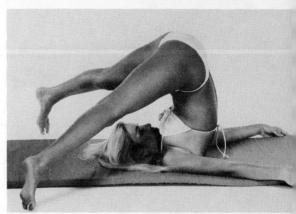

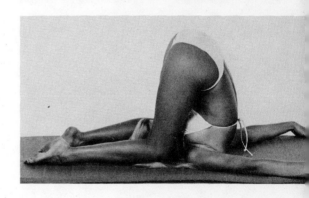

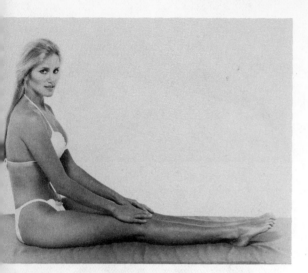

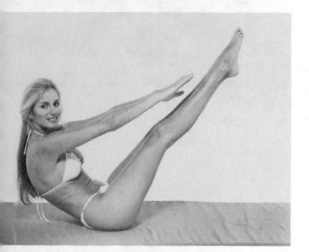

THE JACKKNIFE

There are two very good variations of this exercise. Both of them are excellent for building flexibility in the abdomen and for gaining a sense of balance, using your buttocks as the fulcrum. The first variation: Lie on your back on the floor, stretched completely out, as though you are Superman flying upside down. Start by sitting on the floor with your legs out straight in front of you, hands under your hamstrings. Now, keeping your back straight and making all movements at the abdominals, bring yor legs off the floor and bring your arms out straight to touch your feet. This is not a difficult exercise to do, until you realize that we want you to hold it for a count of fifteen. It will take some practice to learn to balance yourself on your buttocks, and you can practice this one by doing simple toe-touches, which are similar, although they are performed in a different plane. Or, the other alternative, until you get your balance down, is to enlist the aid of your lover to serve as a spotter for you. The object is to be able to do ten of these in a very smooth, flowing motion.

Benefits: Increases flexibility in the lower back, perfects balance, and stretches backs of legs.

HIGH-PITCHED PELVIS

This is a good Sexercise for the all-important pelvic area. Lie on your back and make inverted "V's" with your arms and legs, placing palms and soles flat on the floor under you: They'll serve as your foundations. Now, slowly and carefully, lift the hips and back off the floor and hold yourself in that position for a count of ten. You should be off the floor by about eight inches, and your trunk should be parallel to the floor. Don't expect to get this one down perfectly on the first try. Your arms will likely be much weaker than your muscles in the legs in trying to raise yourself evenly. Don't get discouraged; just keep working on it. Repeat this one three times at first, with a goal of ten times once you've mastered it.

Benefits: Builds strength in the arms, legs, back and shoulders, as well as in the all-important pelvic area.

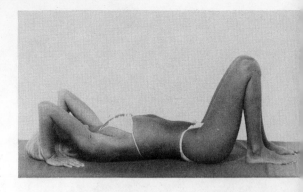

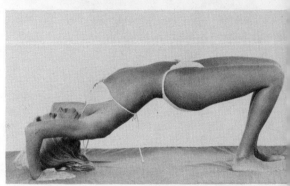

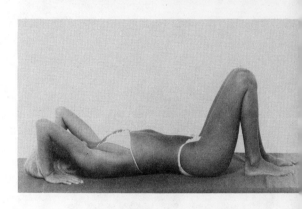

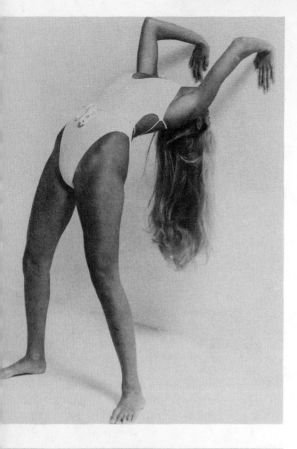

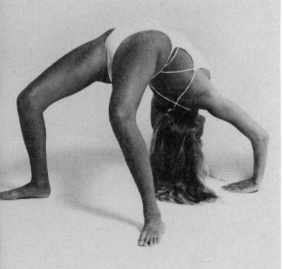

SPIDERWOMAN

I'm using the term "Spider*woman*" because of my sex, but males doing these exercises can certainly refer to it as "Spider-*man*." I've often fantasized about the number of positions for sex available to a contortionist. Most of us aren't as flex-muscled as a contortionist, but once you've mastered this Sexercise, I'm sure it will suggest many possibilities to you in your future lovemaking. Stand with your back to a wall, then walk away from the wall, three lengths of your foot. Now bend over backward very carefully (you might want to use a spotter to help you master this one), placing your palms on the wall while you look toward the ceiling; begin to walk your way down the wall, an inch at a time. This Sexercise is certainly not suggested for anyone with a bad back, and even people with normally good backs may encounter some resistance from this one if they are not properly warmed up. If your back begins to bother you, stop and go on to another Sexercise. Eventually you should be able to walk all the way down the wall — and then walk all the way back up. You're not expected to do this one on the first try, of course. When you do have it down, however, repeat it five times. If, while doing it, you become stalled and cannot get back up the wall, merely allow yourself to roll toward one side or the other, gently dropping to the floor.

Benefits: Strengthens arms and legs, and adds tremendous flexibility to the back.

KNOTTY

This one, done correctly, could get you a good job in a circus. No, seriously, it is less difficult than it looks once you get everything coordinated. Start by sitting on the floor. Now, cock your left leg under you, and bring your right foot up over the knee of the left leg. Your right arm can support you from behind, using your left hand to set your right leg into its proper position. Now, bring your left arm up over your right leg, grasping the right ankle, and bring your right arm behind you, and at the same time, turn your head to look over your right shoulder. You'll feel your muscles stretching in unusual directions. This builds excellent flexibility. Hold fifteen seconds, and then reverse to other side. Repeat five times to a side.

Benefits: Stretches and loosens muscles of the arms and legs.

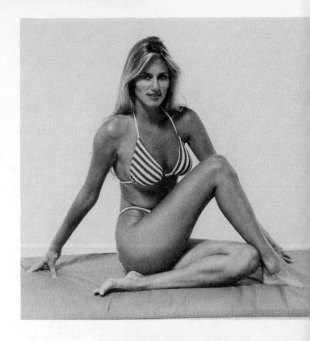

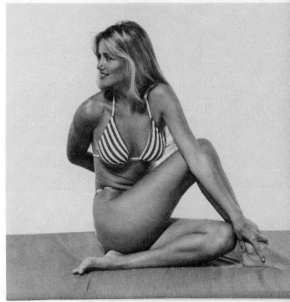

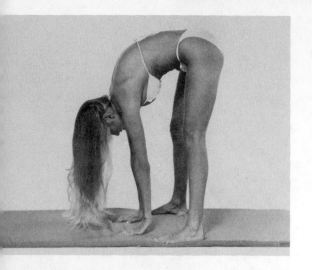

TRIPOD

Stand up straight. Now, bending at the waist, plant your palms on the floor in front of you, on either side of your feet. Now, holding that position, slowly raise your right leg behind you, keeping it straight. Your forehead should then be brought forward to touch lightly to your left leg. Hold for five seconds, and return to the position with both hands and feet on the floor. Then alternate by raising the left leg. Repeat five times to a leg.

Benefits: Stretches back of legs, adds flexibility to hips.

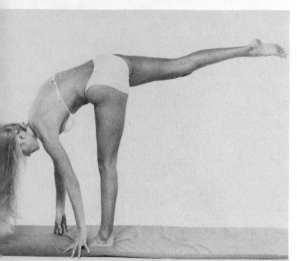

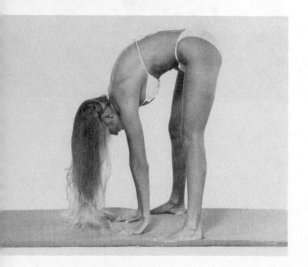

PROPELLERS

This one simulates the action of airplane propellers, and it takes quite a bit of coordination. Lie on your back. You can place your hands under your hips for support if you wish. Now, with your feet out straight, raise them about one foot off the floor and spread them about two feet apart. Now, spin your lower legs in a clockwise direction, at a very steady speed. Do this for fifty repetitions, clockwise, and then, without resting, reverse direction and do fifty more reps. Now, again without resting, raise your thighs to a position perpendicular to the floor, and again begin your clockwise spinning; then reverse, and do fifty reps for each direction. Drop your legs slowly back into the starting position and take a deep breath.

Benefits: Builds strength in the upper legs, lower back and hips, and flexibility in the lower legs.

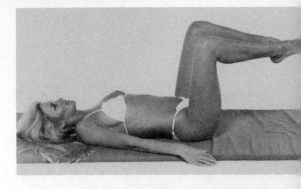

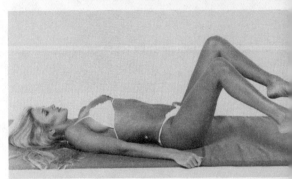

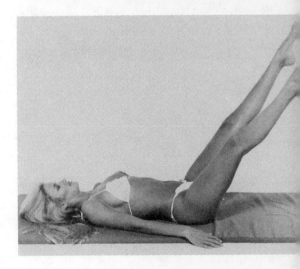

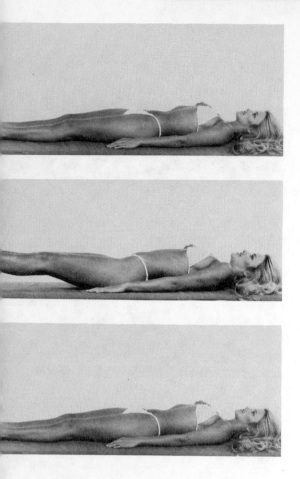

IMMOBILITY

This one is a variation of some of the other Sexercises you have done — simple, yet difficult. Lie down on your back. Keep your legs straight and together, and place your arms at your sides, with your hands under your buttocks for support. Now, with your legs straight and together, lift them four inches off the floor — and hold them there. That's it. Really simple, right? So what's the big trick, huh? Just keep holding them there. Hold them for as long as you can. Just keep holding them there. Now you're begining to see what I mean by it being difficult at the same time, right? You'll begin to feel your muscles protesting, but continue to hold your legs up there. It is becoming more difficult all the time, but you can do it, right? Just keep it up. When you absolutely can't handle it anymore, lower them, pause for thirty seconds, and do it again. You'll feel Immobility working on your thighs, your lower back, and your abdominals. Repeat five times, holding as long as you can.

Benefits: Builds strength in the upper leg, stomach and lower back.

THE SWOOPING HAWK

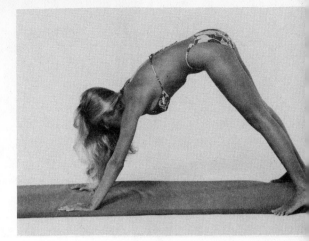

There is a beauty to the movements of the human body that is unique. Watch slow-motion films of a good skier flashing down through a field of moguls. Such beautiful body movements are a combination of many smaller movements made in concert with a set purpose or goal. This Sexercise is a combination of small movements that create a unique exercise, while introducing flexibility workouts into numerous parts of the body. Start by assuming a standard push-up position, but allow the chest to lie on the floor, while the buttocks are raised. In the first segment of this sequence, push with the arms, not unlike the standard push-up. Get ready, and push the arms straight. Keep the legs parallel to the floor, though, and arch the small of the back, throwing back your head at the same time. Before the momentum of the movement can be lost, roll into a movement throwing the hips up toward the ceiling, while keeping the legs straight. Form a mountain with your body, and as you top out, go back toward the floor in a swooping motion; drop your chest toward the floor like a hawk swooping down on its prey. Go right back into the exercise, however, keeping the movement fluid and strong. Do the Swooping Hawk five times, with an ultimate goal of doing it twenty times. The advantages for the male who perfects this one are obvious.

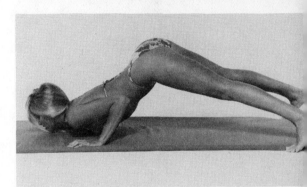

Benefits: Terrific for stretching the front of the body and for flexing the entire spine; strengthens the arms and legs.

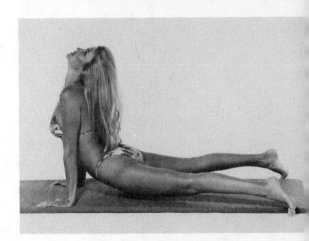

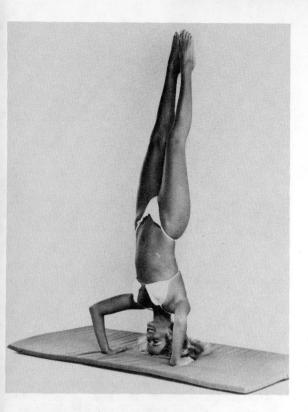

VERTICAL PUSH-UPS

This one is a perfect way to build the arms and sense of balance. Make sure than you do not have shoes on when you do this, or you'll leave marks on the walls. Walk up to bare wall and do a head-stand on the floor, your feet and back up against the wall. Now, this one is going to take a long time to develop properly. You may not be able to do even one when you begin; but, like everything else, if you keep working on it, you'll get quick results. Now that you're comfortable there, attempt to push yourself up off the floor by using just your arms. Keep your body perfectly straight and in contact with the wall. Push as best you can, attempting to work to a straight-arm position. Hold for a second, and slowly return to contact your head to the floor. Then repeat the Sexercise five times.

Benefits: Builds strength in the arms and promotes balance and body awareness.

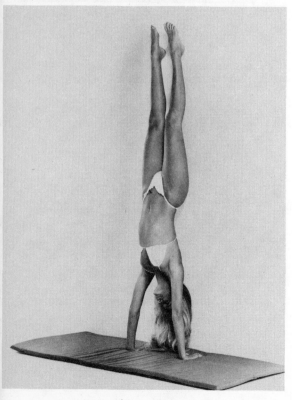

THE REAR-VIEW MIRROR

This is a sort of extreme edition of the toe-touch. Stand up straight and tall. Now, keeping your legs straight and your hips solid, and bending at the waist, reach down and grasp your ankles with your hands. But, instead of stopping there, take it one step farther, and bring your head down far enough so that you can see upside down and behind you by looking through the space between your shins. Push your head through as far as it will go. Hold for five seconds, and return to an upright position. Repeat this one twenty times, trying to get a fraction of an inch farther with each dip.

Benefits: Stretches the back of the legs and the lower back, adds flexibility to the hips.

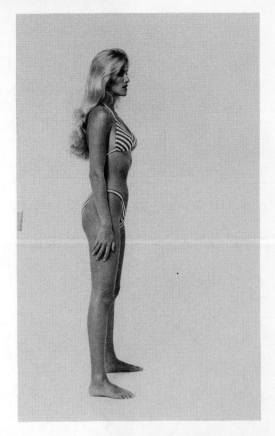

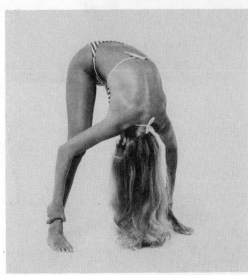

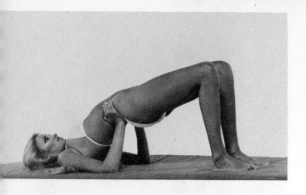

SKY TOWER

Sky Tower provides excellent work for the shoulders and the back, and for working the internal organs. As you reverse the pull of gravity internally, your organs will shift slightly and will be placed into a temporarily relaxed position. Start on your back, arms cocked under your back. Place your hands on your waist to offer a structural support for the building of your tower. Lift your hips off the floor by the support from your hands, and then lift the legs above your head, keeping the legs perfectly straight. So, roll into the position with your legs at a 45-degree angle and hold a second. Then, in a power drive toward the sky, bring your hips and legs into perfectly vertical alignment, forming a tower to the sky, with your shoulders and your arms making a very strong foundation. Hold the position for fifteen seconds; return to floor; repeat ten times.

Benefits: Balance is increased, and strength is built in the legs.

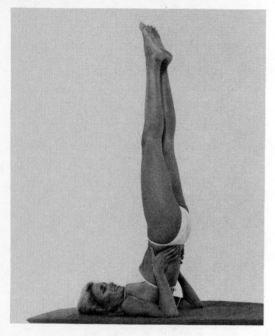

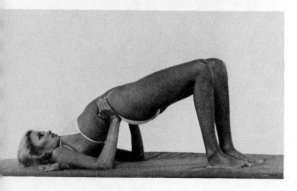

THE DOUBLE DOG

This one would probably be more accurately called the Dog-and-Hydrant, but we'll just call it the Double Dog. It goes one step beyond the Dog in difficulty. Get down on all fours like old Spot would. Keep your back straight; no swayback on this. Your arms and thighs should be perfectly vertical to the floor. Now, without moving anything but the right leg, raise it until it is parallel to the floor, keeping it bent at the knee. Hold the leg there for a second, and then extend it out straight, concentrating on keeping everything else perfectly still. This one is certainly not easy to do, but offers great results. You feel the pull in the muscles along the outside of your buns, and along the entire length of your leg. Hold the position for a count of ten, then bend the leg back, and return to all fours. Now repeat on the other side. You should do this one a total of ten times to the side.

Benefits: Builds strength in the legs.

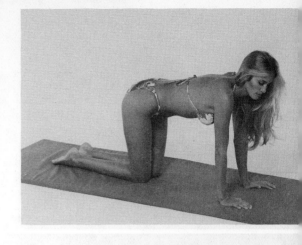

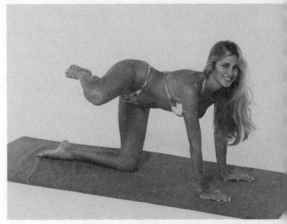

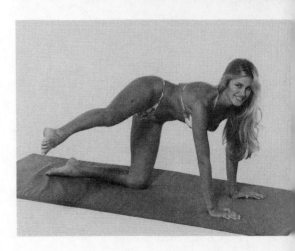

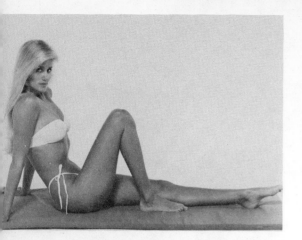

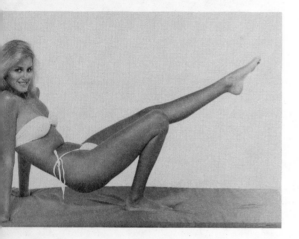

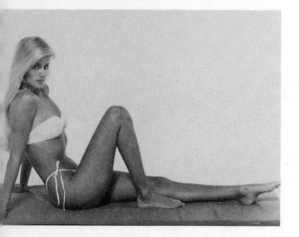

THREE-LEGGED CHAIR

Sit on the floor, your legs out in front of you. Place your palms on the floor at the sides of your hips, directly under your shoulders. Now, bring your right leg up, planting the sole of your foot solidly on the floor at the point where your lower leg is vertical. Keep your left leg out straight. Now, lift your butt off the floor using your arms and your right leg. Raise yourself until your arms are straight. Now, begin scribing a perfect square in the air with your left foot. The square should be about eighteen inches to the side. Make the box ten times, and then bring your left foot down next to your right foot. You now have a four-legged chair. You know, of course, that this is only temporary. Now lift your right leg up, stretch it out straight and make your box ten times on the right. Then do it ten times again with the left, and then ten more times with the right.

Benefits: Builds strength in the arms and legs, and builds flexibility in the legs.

PRO PUSH-UPS

We're not going to make this one as diffi-cult as it was for the Italian Stallion in *"Rocky,"* but this is the Intense Level, and it's a good Sexercise to work on to build your arms, which are one of the most ne-glected regions of development in the aver-age female. Drop into the basic push-up po-sition. Keep your entire body straight, your toes in contact with the floor, and all work coming through your arms. Think of your body as a wooden plank or as a diving board. Now, rather than using both arms to push yourself up and down, balance yourself on your right arm and grasp your right wrist with your left hand. Now, do five push-ups. Then, reverse, putting your right hand around your left wrist, and do five more push-ups. As you become stronger, you can increase the number of push-ups by one ad-ditional push-up per week.

Benefits: Builds tremendous strength in the arms.

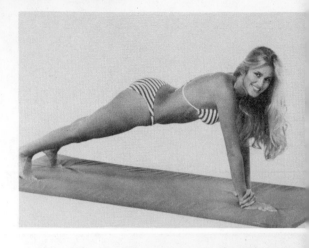

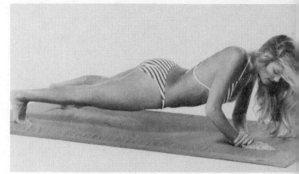

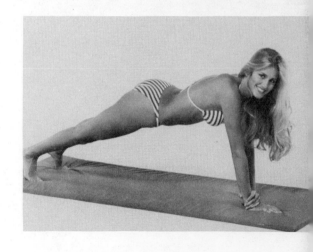

CHAPTER 5

For Women Only

This chapter comes to you after plenty of soul-searching and census-taking. I had originally planned to include it, then I had second thoughts. But I talked to quite a few people — both men and women — and they convinced me that the subject in this chapter definitely deserves attention. It has rarely been touched on.

This is a discussion of the female organs, sex from the woman's side, and exercises to allow the woman to strengthen internal muscles. These muscles allow for more variety and pleasure in lovemaking, for both the woman and her partner.

At first I wanted to include this chapter because, even though a woman might be very well educated, that is no guarantee her education dealt with the organs that make her a woman. Schools have always been reluctant to deal with subjects on sex, for two main reasons. First, the educators were unable to get the information across to the students in a form that the students could understand. The teachers were not specially educated on the subject. Second, the schools' best efforts were short-circuited or stifled by parents, who felt that sex-education classes were akin to taking little kids to a porn-film festival.

Times have not changed. Parents still don't want their children to learn about sex in sex-education classes. Unfortunately, very few children are learning about sex at home. The parents of their parents had the same attitude. They didn't want their children learning about sex, so the situation continues unchanged from one generation to the next. It is a very unhealthy situation, one that feeds upon itself, and that propagates the problem for generations to come. Because children are not getting the sex education they need at home or at school, there has been an incredible rise in teen-age pregnancies.

My feeling, then, is that a discussion of the female sex organs, at least insofar as they can be affected by exercise, is in order. The discussion will not be an anatomy class, and it will not be a strictly sex-education class. Instead, it will be a free-wheeling discussion of some very real considerations for women.

The reason for not having a chapter for men is simply because they have few muscles related to their sex organs that can or would be affected by exercise. Oh, that's not to say that some guys haven't exercised certain muscles in their lower abdomens so that by

contracting them, they can do some tricks, but there are no really significant changes that a man can make to the function of his sex organs. Southside Johnny and the Asbury Jukes sing a song that cautions, "It ain't the meat/It's the motion." And as far as male techniques are concerned, that's pretty much true. Good external moves are what make a male a good lover.

I finally decided that there was absolutely no reason *not* to have a chapter on exercising internally.

A woman has the ability to build up and develop certain muscles that can have a profound affect upon her enjoyment of sex by making her more comfortable. Once developed, they can give her a certain unique control of the direction lovemaking takes. By building up and learning how to control certain muscles, she can add significantly to the enjoyment she and her lover get from making love.

After talking to quite a few people about the concept of the chapter, however, I learned that there was interest from both sexes in this subject. Women were interested because they wanted to know more about improving their ability as lovers. The men I spoke with felt it would be a terrific chapter for them to share with their lovers. They talked of improving their sex by allowing the female to take a more active role.

So it is not without apprehension that I'm including this chapter. I feel it is important, but I think it is equally important for readers to understand why it is here. Some of you will already know much of what I'm about to discuss. Many of you will have had experiences with some of these muscles and will know exactly what I'm talking about, but will not have suspected that there are ways of doing something positive to get more control over them — and to be able to use them in your lovemaking. A few of you may think it's somewhat kinky; I don't think so. It's something that is very much a part of you. Making your body work better in order to more fully enjoy your lovemaking is not one bit weird.

Muscles are muscles. If you believe you should work on your biceps in order to build additional strength and keep off fat, there is no reason to stop there. There are several additional benefits that have nothing to do with sex; for example, strengthening these muscles can make menstrual cramps much less severe, and they can reduce the strain of childbirth.

Let's start with some simple anatomy. Between your neck and your genitals, there are three major and distinct cavities inside your body. You are not merely a big, hollow cavity, with things like a stomach and heart and intestines thrown in there randomly. Instead, you are built like a three-story building; each of the three stories is separate, but connected at certain points, and each has very specific functions.

The top story, called the thoracic cavity, starts at the neck and goes down to the diaphragm, which forms the floor of the top

the back, they are held in by the spine and the back wall of the cavity.

The bottom story is primarily bordered by the walls of the pelvis, and is logically called the pelvic cavity. Here is where we will concentrate in this chapter. The pelvic area contains the kidneys, bladder, prostate, small intestine, the urethra, colon and sex organs.

Most of the organs in the pelvic region are common to the sexes because they have identical functions. The differences, or course, lie in the sex organs, primarily in the uterus of the woman and the scrotum and penis of the male.

Our concern here is with the female and

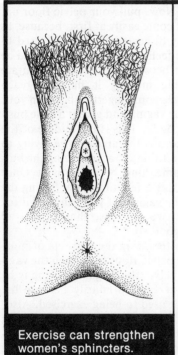

Exercise can strengthen women's sphincters.

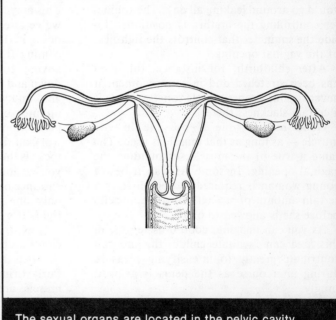

The sexual organs are located in the pelvic cavity, along with the kidneys and intestines.

story and the roof of the second story. The diaphragm is level with the ribs and, in fact, the ribs serve as walls of that story. The upper story contains the heart, the lungs, and air and food passages.

The middle story is the abdominal cavity. The abdominal cavity starts at a point directly below the ribs and extends to the top of the pelvic region. The abdominal cavity contains the stomach, pancreas, large intestine, the liver, and the like. The abdominal or "stomach" muscles, the ones that look like a washboard in bodybuilders, hold the internal organs inside the cavity, while from

that portion of her anatomy at the bottom of the pelvic cavity. It is known as the pelvic diaphragm or the pelvic floor.

The pelvic diaphragm is a series of large, flat muscles stretched across the pelvis, from wall to wall. You can locate them easily. Stand up straight, legs together. Now, change your legs to a position where your feet are 18 inches apart. Your pelvic diaphragm is what prevented all of your internal organs from falling through the bottom of your pelvis and onto the floor when you spread your legs. To better understand the pelvic diaphragm, cup your hands in front of you. That, essentially, is the shape of the diaphragm. It holds your abdominal organs in place and, since it consists of muscles, it can be strengthened.

Now, while still looking at your cupped hands, note where your two hands meet — at the little fingers of both hands. In the female, at approximately the three knuckles of the little fingers, there are openings. If your fingertips are the front of the pelvic diaphragm, the three openings from front to rear (literally) are the urethra, vagina and rectum.

Each of the three openings is held closed by sphincter muscles, which are muscles in a band or circle that can open by relaxing and close by contracting. Without the sphincter, you'd go around leaking all day. The sphincter controlling the urethra is positioned inside the sphincter that controls the tightness of the vaginal opening.

After childbirth, for instance, this area has been stretched and in some women, it never regains proper muscle tone, so there is a certain slackness there.

Good muscle tone is possible in any muscle — as long as that muscle is used. The same it true of the muscle surrounding the vaginal opening. In some African tribes, a young woman is required to demonstrate a certain amount of strength in these muscles before she is allowed to marry.

As you can imagine, good muscle tone in this area can facilitate childbirth, and can contribute greatly to intensifying pleasure during intercourse as the penis is gripped snugly.

You can get a good idea of the strength you have in your genital muscles by sitting in a bath and inserting your finger into your vagina. Now, attempt to close upon your finger. If you can't feel any pressure being exerted, you've got a lot of work to do there. Some women have developed this region to the point where they can almost trap their lover's penis inside.

These muscles and the muscles that control the walls of the vagina contract spasmodically during and immediately following orgasm, and many of the body's muscles that work involuntarily can be trained to work voluntarily, also. Imagine how you can improve your sex life if you can gain control of these muscles and develop their strength.

There are certain exercises you can do that will strengthen and tone your pelvic and lower abdominal muscles so that you can really tighten up and make good use of that muscle tone and muscle control. The first step is to become familiar with the feeling of the muscles involved. By becoming attuned to them, you can better recognize the part they play, and you can more easily practice getting control of them.

The two primary movements are raising the pelvic floor and tightening the sphincter at the mouth of the vagina. Although doing exercises with these muscles may be unusual for you, they are in no way dangerous.

Lie on your back and divorce your attention from anything else going on around you. Think only of your pelvic region and how it feels. Now, pull your pelvic floor up. This may not come easily at first, because, as we've already discussed, you aren't used to doing it. The feeling of movement should be coming from between your legs. If you are having trouble making it happen, reach down and place your fingertips between your anus and your vagina and give it a little push up into your body. This is the middle of the pelvic floor and is the area you're trying to work on. Don't think that squeezing the buttocks is the same thing, because it isn't. Once you've done this a few times, try flexing the entrance of the vagina. If you can hold it for only one or two seconds, that's quite all right. It's a good start.

Now, try alternating the two sets of muscles. Flex the pelvic floor first, then the vagina, then the pelvic floor again. This may be fairly tiring at first, primarily because the muscles aren't used to being exercised. Also, because they're out of shape, you are having to work doubly hard to exert voluntary control over them.

Now, for another warm-up exercise, and as a means of familiarizing yourself with another movement, place your hand over the pubic bone, and try to fight against gravity by bringing the birth canal up to your hand. Don't move your hips or flex your buttocks when you are doing it. All effort should be internal. If you manage to do it, hold a few seconds and then release. Note particularly the sensation as the pelvic floor relaxes. Try to slacken it a little more; in fact, try to release all tension. Do only two or three in succession before resting.

Once you've mastered an awareness of these muscles, you can exercise them from virtually any position, which is terrific because you can work exercises into your everyday life without causing a sensation.

Eventually, you'll want to bring into play neighboring muscle groups, such as the buttocks, inner thighs and abdominals, so that you are exercising the entire pelvic region. You will soon see the inter-relationship between the muscle groups.

Your goal is to do your contractions in sets of five, with a rest between sets. You don't have to go beyond five reps in a set. What you can do, however, is intersperse sets of five throughout your day until you are doing about fifty contractions a day. Hold each contraction for five seconds.

A few words about the abdominal muscles before we get into the exercises that are designed for building this often overlooked region of the body. The abdominal muscles are certainly much easier to see, and their importance to posture and general body strength is profound. The abdominals are often referred to as the stomach muscles. They are the muscles most directly affected by doing sit-ups.

A friend of mine who runs marathons tells me that strong stomach muscles are extremely important in the last five or six miles of a marathon. As the body tires, it tends to weaken all over, and one's stride can be shortened. But the abdominal muscles, if they are properly developed, can contribute greatly to keeping the upper body straight and fluid.

Many people let their abdominals go to pot — literally. The typical potbelly is a person (either man or woman) who allows his or her abdominals to weaken; they stretch and get slack when weakened, and the body begins spilling over the belt buckle. This can cause many problems, including lower-back pain, improper tilt of the pelvis, and poor breathing.

Weak abdominals can also seriously affect lovemaking. Ladies, if you've ever been lying on your back and attempted to raise your head to kiss your lover and felt a quivering in the stomach, it was likely not a quivering of emotion, but rather a quivering due to weak abdominal muscles; hold that position long enough, and the quivering would soon turn to spasms.

For men, the abdominal muscles are extremely important, because once your lover gets into a pumping rhythm, it is frequently the abdominals that are doing the work. If they weaken quickly and thus cause him to lose his concentration, the enjoyment of lovemaking could be ruined.

The easiest and most basic approach to improving the abdominals is to do a regimen of sit-ups — and there are many variations on the basic sit-up. I've put together some exercises that I use almost daily and, that I think you'll agree, are perfect for directly working the corresponding sex parts we're concerned with here.

As with all the other Sexercises, you should do these regularly but patiently. Don't try to do everything at once: That's the best way to turn yourself off to Sexercise. Start by doing limited repetitions, and establish a foundation; build upon that.

Now, without further foreplay, let's get into the Sexercises "For Women Only."

THE ELECTRIC CHAIR

Sit upright in a chair that has armrests. Place your forearms on the armrests. Now, raise yourself off the seat of the chair using only your arms. Feel your abdominal muscles tightening? Your abdominals, especially those circling your navel, are pulling upward. Hold this position for a count of five, and then settle back into the chair.

Now that you know the feeling you're working for, let's add some other exercises. The next time you lift up, keep your buttocks lightly touching the chair seat, and tighten the muscles around the vagina; attempt to "suck" them up as high as possible. At the same time, try tightening your buttocks.

Now, when you do the exercise this time, try holding yourself up off the seat for a count of ten; on each odd number you count, tighten the muscles around the vagina and the buttocks, and on each even number relax both the vagina and buttocks. It may be difficult at first to do this more than one or two times, but keep working on it until you get to the point where you can do ten of these. You can do this exercise while sitting at home watching TV, or you can do it at the office when everyone is looking the other way.

I call it The Electric Chair because once I became adept at doing it, I experienced some electric arousal. Don't worry, if this happens; it lets you know that you are using your muscles.

THE SQUEEZE

This is one that you can start at home, and once you get it down, you can do it anywhere and absolutely no one will know you're going at it.

At home, lie down on your back in a quiet room. Now, relaxing yourself as best you can, suck in the pelvic floor and draw the muscles upward. Pretend that there is something inside you (your lover?), and gently squeeze. It is important that you do not use any other muscles. Don't squeeze with your legs or your buttocks; use only the muscles around your vagina. Hold the squeeze for a count of three and then release. The object is not to develop jaws of steel, but merely to get to know what muscles you have there, to learn to control them and to become sensitive to them. This should ultimately be one of the easiest exercises you can do. Repeat it a half-dozen times that first session on the floor, keeping in mind that the object is to learn *control*. Strength will come as you repeat the exercise.

If you think you need to do a few more sessions at home on the floor, go right ahead. Once you have mastered it, however, you can do this exercise anywhere, at any time, in any position, and no one is going to know you're doing it.

I put together — in a matter of seconds — a list of places I practice this one: while cooking, in elevators, waiting in lines, while brushing my teeth, while sitting at a stop light in my car, while talking on the phone, while luxuriating in bed the first thing in the morning before getting up, while waiting for a waiter at a restaurant, at parties, at concerts, while putting on some makeup. The opportunities are endless.

Once you have it perfected, try it out on your lover, and see what kind of reaction you receive.

THE PROGRESSION

This one starts off solo and progresses to being done with your lover.

Having gotten a feel for the action of the muscle around your vagina, you should now start to perfect it. Lie down on your bed, spread your legs and relax. Take a finger and carefully insert it. Now, in a rapid, machine-gun fashion, constrict the walls quickly for as long as you can. Typically, you'll feel pressure on your finger at first and, then, as the muscle tires, the pressure will diminish. When it gives out, relax a few minutes, and then do it again.

If you faithfully do this exercise, two things should happen: You'll begin to be able to grip your finger more firmly on the first contraction, and you'll be able to keep the contractions going longer. Once you feel comfortable with your strength and length of constrictions, it's time to get a little assistance from your lover.

When you and your partner are comfortable, explain to him what you are attempting to do. He'll be very interested in helping with the exercise, if he's any kind of lover. He'll have to be very cooperative, because once he enters you, he's got to stay quiet and relaxed on you.

When he's in the lovemaking position, begin the controlled contractions. If you were having success contracting your finger, it should be infinitely easier — and more fun — contracting your lover's penis, because his penis is much larger than your finger. As you perfect it, your lover's going to have to exert a great deal of self-control to lie on you quietly while you do this, because it can be exquisitely stimulating.

This exercise will certainly enhance a lovemaking session for both of you.

HAND JOB

This exercise can — and should — be done twice a day, the most convenient times being when you wake in the morning, and before you retire in the evening. It can be done most conveniently in bed, and it takes only a few minutes. It concentrates on control.

Lie on your back, and prop your head up with a pillow so that you can easily see your stomach. It will be more difficult for you to see your progress if you are fleshy in the tummy; the more flesh you have there, the more difficult it is to see your muscles work. In Hand Job the goal is to relax your legs and your buttocks so that you don't cheat by moving yourself in the pelvic area with anything but your sphincter muscles.

Contract the muscle around the vagina and see if there is any response in the belly muscles. There may not be anything noticeable. So now comes the hands-on policy. Gently place your hand flat on the flesh just below your navel. Try to squeeze your muscles directly under the hand. Now, make it a little more difficult, and move the hand over to the side. Try to move the muscles that are inside yourself and under your hand.

Move your hand again. And react there by making muscles under your hand. This sounds relatively difficult, but with practice it becomes quite a good workout that will give you incredible control, and that will also prepare you well for childbirth.

TILT!

By developing strength and flexibility in the pelvic area, you can relieve stiffness and backache, while greatly improving your ability to enjoy sex.

Perhaps the practitioner who best exemplifies the possibilities of pelvic tilt is the belly dancer. She makes strong, sure moves by allowing the pelvis to flow forward and back, and from side to side.

The pelvis is held up in the front by the abdominal muscles, which is why people with big, fat stomachs also tend to exhibit bad posture: Instead of their abdominals working to hold the pelvis up in front, the weight of the slack muscles pushes it down. In the back, the pelvis is pulled down by the buttocks. If both abdominal muscles and buttocks are toned and firm, there is a dynamic balance to the pelvis, and you have proper posture and strength in the pelvic area.

There are several ways to do the Tilt; here's the easiest: Lie on your back on a floor, without padding between the hard floor and you, because we want you to attempt to flatten the small of your back against the floor; insert your hand between your back and the floor to make sure your back is flat.

When you are on your back, bring your knees up, your soles flat on the floor, your heels touching your buttocks. Place your hands lightly in the hollow of the small of your back, because the object is to press your back onto the floor, squeezing your hands. Now, breathe out, and at the same time tighten your buttocks and abdomen and hold them. This action should have pressed your back down against the floor. Make sure while you are doing this that you don't raise your buttocks off the floor.

Repeat this one a dozen times, holding it to a count of five each time. A variation of Tilt can be done while on your hands and knees, and is very similar to the yoga exercise known as The Cat.

THE SPREAD

The most common position a woman takes during lovemaking is one in which she spreads her legs to accept her lover. This is not a position that you commonly practice during the average day, unless you are a gymnast or a ballet dancer.

It is very frustrating to be making love and suddenly be seized with aches and pains in your legs, as a result of their being spread uncomfortably wide or from being spread so long that they begin to hurt. It is a discomfort women do not frequently go around talking about, but it is certainly not uncommon.

I encourage you to do exercises from the Casual, Intimate and Intense sections that stress flexibility and strength in the legs, especially those that stress benefits to the inner thigh.

You can work little exercises into your everyday life that will greatly benefit your groin and inner thigh area. For example, when you are sitting watching TV or reading, why not be on the floor in a Butterfly or lotus position? Gravity will gently stretch your muscles and will make those previously uncomfortable positions not only tolerable, but enjoyable.

CHAPTER 6
Sexercises for Lovers

Although sex is an activity best enjoyed with another, exercising is something that you must do for yourself. It is ultimately an individual activity. No one can do your exercising for you. No one can cover for you if you ignored a certain exercise.

There is a popular bumper sticker in auto racing that reads: "When the green flag drops, the bullshit stops." What it means is that you can blow your horn and brag all you want, but if you haven't got the goods when the time comes, you're going to make a fool of yourself, for all the world to see. It is also like that in aerobic, non-team sports — tennis, running, racquetball, cycling, etc. You practice your sport, and then you compete against other people who practice it, or you put yourself up against the clock — and you either make it or you don't.

Exercising is more philosophical and more private. You aren't expected to enter a contest where you challenge someone to doing the maximum number of sit-ups in an hour. Exercising is something that you do for yourself and, indirectly, for your loved ones; you have no one else to whom you must answer. You can do your exercising in private, and if you decide to test yourself at some point by seeing how many sit-ups you can perform in an hour, that's all well and good. There won't be a crowd of fifty thousand spectators munching popcorn and drinking beer out of waxed cups, and Howard Cosell won't be pushing a mike into your face and asking you mile-long questions that you're too winded to answer anyway. Your cheering section will be your determination, your personal integrity.

Although it breaks the mold I've been trying to establish with this book, there will be some of you who want to occasionally challenge yourself, to see where you are in your fitness, and I applaud you for that. I also set up private goals for a specific exercising session, and then I bust ass to reach that goal. It can be fun, and even if you have never been competitive in sports or physical activities, it brings out personality traits that you did not even suspect existed. There is a certain tenaciousness that emerges in some people that is quite interesting. The seemingly meek are often the most iron-willed when it comes to personal challenges and achieving personal goals.

But, for the most part, I like to be philosophical about my exercising. By that, I mean that I like to allow exercising to become an integral part of my life and my life philosophy; as such, it does not in any way intrude upon my life. Instead, exercise is a part of my life, a reflection of myself. As far as how I like to do my exercises, you could say that I'm pretty flexible (no pun, really).

As I've stated before, there are some days when I enjoy nothing more than putting on some good music and slipping into a body stocking, getting down on the rug and easing into an hour-long exercising session. I'll gradually build up until I'm loose enough to do any exercise; then I'll cool down and finish with a relaxing shower. This workout can really enliven me, and puts a real edge on my day.

There are other times when I enjoy exercising with a group. I am almost always involved in an exercising group that meets regularly. I find that although my individual exercising is spontaneous and extremely enjoyable, it is also valuable to have certain times of the week set aside when I *know* I'm going to be at an exercise class. I have something to look forward to all day.

Exercising classes can be a lot of fun. You feel part of a movement (literally), you meet some very nice people who share your interests in fitness, and it is a very pleasant social situation. Just be careful not to get into an exercising group that is beyond your current ability; you don't want to be turned off because the class intimidates you.

There is a third way of exercising that I especially enjoy and that is not practiced very much — Sexercise with your lover.

In most sports and activities, males and females don't compete against each other, except on a low-key level. We are, after all, somewhat different anatomically, and we have different capacities. Males have a higher percentage of their body weight in muscle than women, while women have a higher percentage body fat. So, if a male and a female start participating in a sport and are on the same ability level, they will likely progress at different rates. Of course, sometimes a woman is an exceptional athlete and will outshine the man. It is not uncommon to see two lovers running together or cycling together or doing a Parcourse together. But they're doing it together for recreation, not competition. In every sport, with the exception of long-distance swimming (where body fat is crucial), men will outperform women, all things being equal.

There is a physical activity where both lovers can be fairly even, however, and that is in doing exercise programs together. The exercises in this chapter are designed to accommodate lovers by allowing them to work with and against each other at the same level. Some of the exercises call for using your lover's body to provide resistance, while other exercises use him to complement your own.

You never know where these exercises will lead, either. Although I appear in these photographs wearing some clothes, I enjoy doing these exercises in the nude, too. They are rather stimulating, and fun, while beneficial for your physical health.

I've planned the chapter on Sexersaage to follow this one, because after a heated session of "Sexercise with Your Lover," you may need a good massage that brings you through recovery from sex, or that sends you into another sexual episode. Or you may want to give one to your lover. Everything, you see, interrelates.

So, rather than going to the movies or to a show or to dinner, why not stay in for an exercise session? You never know what will come up.

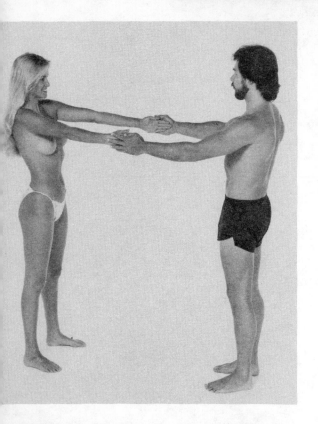

PEC PERKS

This one builds strength in the pectoral muscles, those that go across the chest. Stand facing each other, about four feet apart. Now, extend your arms in front of yourselves, palms together. Your lover should then place the palms of his hands on top of each of your hands, so that he has made a "hand sandwich." Now, while he offers some resistance, try to smoothly separate your hands. Work against the resistance he is offering until your hands are about two feet apart; then have him put his hands inside yours, and have him apply resistance against your attempts to bring your hands back together. Do Pec Perks ten times, and then you do the same for him.

Benefits: Strengthens the pectorals and arms.

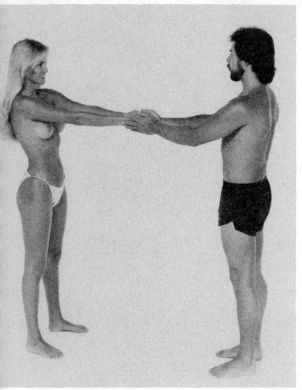

TUG-OF-WAR

Stand facing each other. Now, you take one step to your left, and then one step forward. Both of you are now side-by-side, looking in opposite directions. Place the outside of your feet against each other for support, and grasp hands nearest each other. Now, smoothly and slowly, begin alternating pulling against resistance. You pull first, while your lover offers resistance. Do it for about a minute. Then let him pull against your resistance. It's a sort of mini-tug-of-war, and it can be a lot of fun. When you've done it ten times each, switch sides and start all over with the other arms.

Benefits: Builds arm and leg strength, and promotes a better sense of balance.

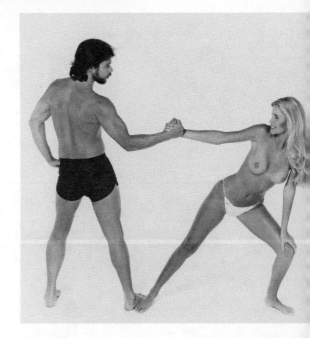

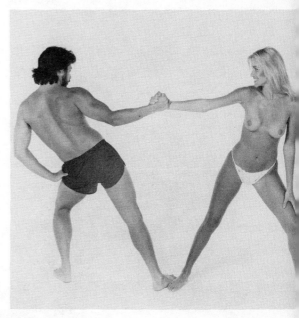

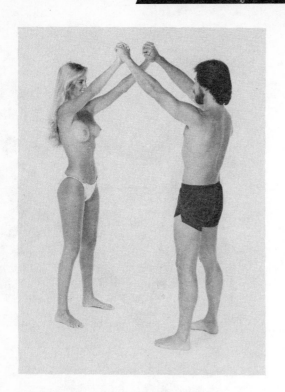

REACH STRETCH

Stand facing each other. Join hands. Now, in the same movement, dip forward slightly to the right while bringing your arms up. Your lover should be doing the same on his side. Offer resistance to each other. You should be bending at the knees. Hold for a count of five and return to your starting position. Then, do the same movement to the left. Offer resistance so that as you go down and forward, you feel as though your arms are engaged with a spring that's capable of bouncing you back. Repeat ten times to the side.

Benefits: Stretches the front of the body, and builds strength in the legs.

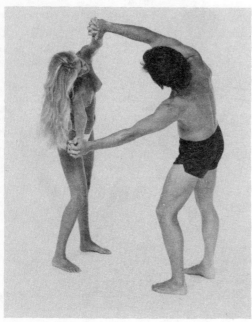

THE TUNNEL

Stand back-to-back. Both of you bend at the waist, allowing your hands to swing down loosely. When your chests are parallel to the floor, swing your arms between your legs, ultimately joining hands under your buttocks. Now, with hands joined, gently and smoothly take turns pulling each other toward the tunnel you've formed. Don't pull too hard and don't jerk your partner. Be very gentle so that you are stretching your back muscles, and not straining them. Pull your partner toward you twenty times, and then slowly return to your starting position.

Benefits: Stretches the back, and increases flexibility in the legs and buttocks.

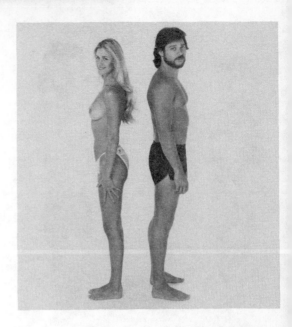

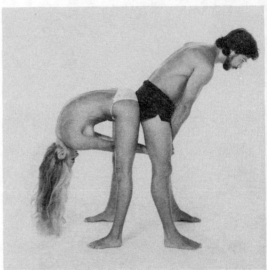

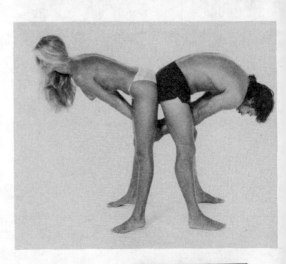

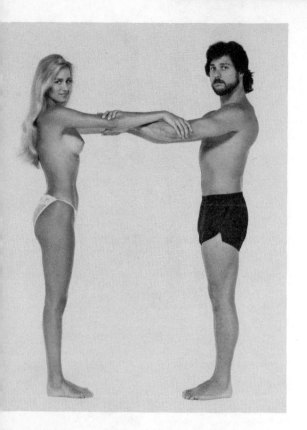

STEREO SQUATS

Stand facing each other and grasp each other's elbows. Now, keeping your feet together amd your heels planted firmly on the floor, bend at the knees and go into a squat, getting down as far as you comfortably can. Hold for ten seconds when you've bottomed out, and then come back up, repeating ten times. You can vary this a bit by coming in a little closer together and taking turns squatting; the partner who remains standing performs the role of a balance bar.

Benefits: Strengthens the legs and increases sense of balance.

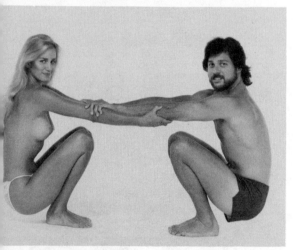

HUMAN BAR

Stand facing each other at a distance equal to the length of your leg if it were extended straight toward your partner, which it will be. Have your partner act as a human ballet bar. Extend your right leg out straight to him and let him cup your heel in his hand, supporting its weight. Your leg should be parallel to the floor. Now, balancing yourself on your left leg, bend forward at the waist and, keeping your back straight, touch your nose to your knee. Repeat five times, then change legs. When you are finished, you can serve as the human ballet bar for your partner.

Benefits: Adds flexibility to the hips, stretches and strengthens the legs.

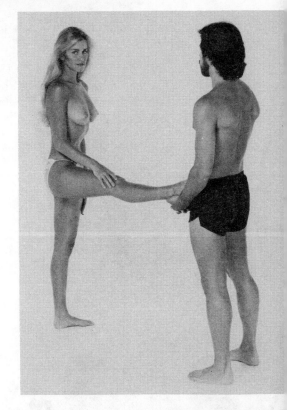

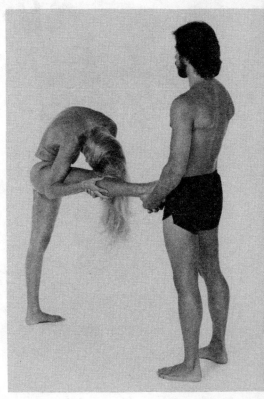

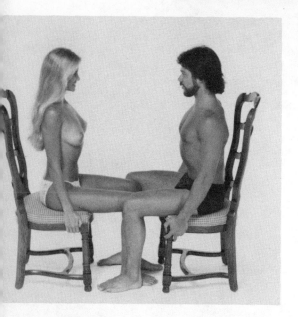

KNEE KNOCKS

Sit on straight-back chairs facing each other, very close. One of you should start by placing your knees inside the other's knees. Now, attempt to separate your knees while your partner applies pressure with his knees to keep them together. Then, put your knees outside his, and press your knees together against resistance from his. Now, have him do the same sequence against your knees. Since he will usually be stronger, you can use your hands on your knees to add resistance. Do this one fifteen times each.

Benefits: Strengthens the thighs.

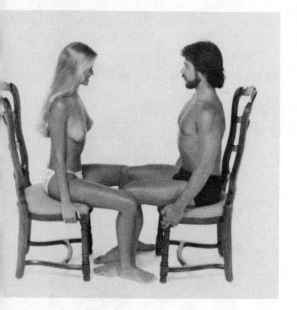

ROLL OVER

Stand back-to-back and interlock arms at the elbows. Now, with your parter taking his turn first, very slowly have him bend forward. This movement will pick you up and off the ground. During the process, you will feel your back bend and the front of your body stretch. All movements should be made slowly and under control, and as soon as you reach a point where this becomes uncomfortable for you, have your lover stop. Pause there a moment and then allow him to lower you back down. When you touch back down, continue the movement by pulling him up on your back, also going very slowly. The secret for you doing this comfortably is to use his weight to your advantage. Keep your legs straight and firmly planted. The person going up at the time should remain completely relaxed so as to make the lift easier on the partner on the bottom. The Roll Over can be repeated five times per partner.

Benefits: Provides terrific stretching for the front of the body, and builds muscles in the leg when you're doing the lifting.

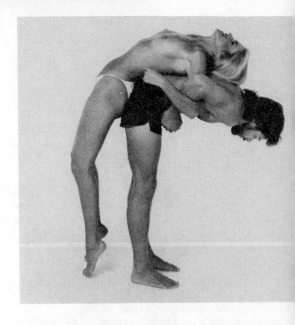

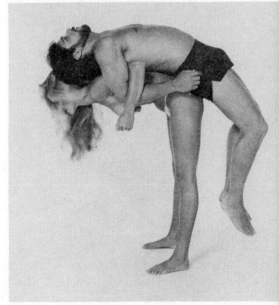

THE ELEVATOR

Stand back-to-back and interlock arms at elbows. Press backs together. It is best to do this and other Sexercises without shoes; your bare feet will grip better, especially if the floor is not covered with a rug. Now, using only your legs, begin to lower yourselves in unison until your buns touch the floor. Once you have made contact with the floor, again using only your legs for elevation, stand back up. Of course, the slower you do this, the better it is for you, because it more thoroughly works the muscles. Repeat The Elevator ten times.

Benefits: Builds strength and tone in the legs.

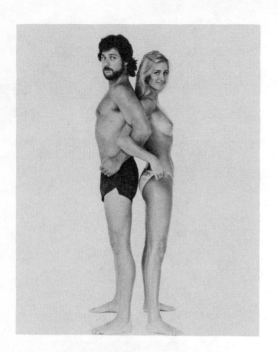

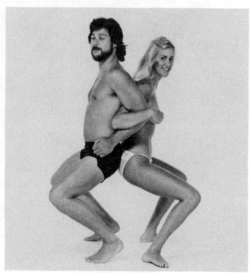

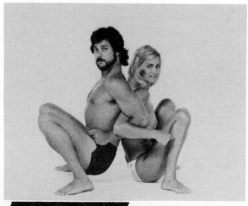

TAFFY PULL

Sit down on the floor facing each other. Spread your legs as far as they'll go, bringing the soles of your respective feet together. Join hands in the middle, getting a good grip. Now, take turns pulling one another toward the middle of the space between you. If you are pulling, pull until you are on your back and your partner is nose-to-the-floor. Then allow him to pull you back up and forward until your nose is on the floor and he is lying with his back on the floor behind him. It is very similar to a seesaw effect. Do this one ten times per person. As you get stronger, you can make the Taffy Pull do even more for you by having the person being pulled offering some resistance.

Benefits: Stretches legs and groin area, and strengthens arms.

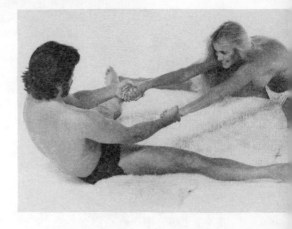

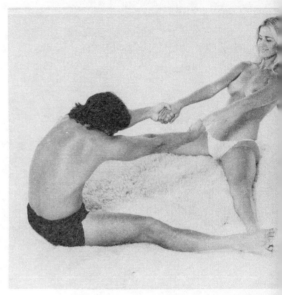

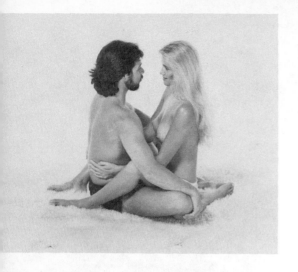

BACK DROP

Sit down on the floor facing each other. Get as close as you can. Your partner should wrap his legs around your hips, and you should wrap your legs around his waist. Now, you wrap your hands around his waist, also, and allow him to drop backward toward the floor, your hands providing a support for his back so that he does not go back too fast. Once he has touched his head to the floor behind him, help him come back up. Now, he can do the same for you. Continue alternating until each of you has done it ten times. Be sure to give as much support as you can, so that there is not a great deal of strain to either of you as you drop back.

Benefits: Stretches the front of the body and builds strength in the back and hips.

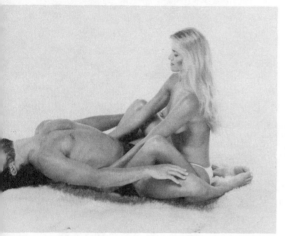

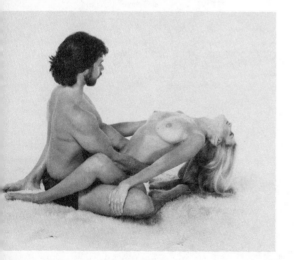

THE PEACOCK

Lie down on the floor, facing each other, but instead of doing Back Drop face-to-face, do it face-to-feet. Get as close as you can. Now, since you are face-to-face, that means you are on your sides, and you therefore have an "up" leg and a "down" leg. Using your "up" hand, grasp your partner's "up" ankle and lift it, extending your arm upward until it becomes straight. Then return your lover's leg. Repeat ten times, then roll over and do it from the opposite arm and leg, still facing each other. What you have, in effect, is a human Nautilus machine. If you are somewhat less developed in the arms than your male partner, and realizing that his legs are probably heavier to lift than yours, you can help him by adding resistance in your leg as he attempts to raise it. And he can help you by lightening his leg so you don't have to struggle too much at first. Eventually, you'll be strong enough to lift it easily. It is also fun to do this exercise nude and let it go where it will once you're properly warmed up.

Benefits: Strengthens the arms.

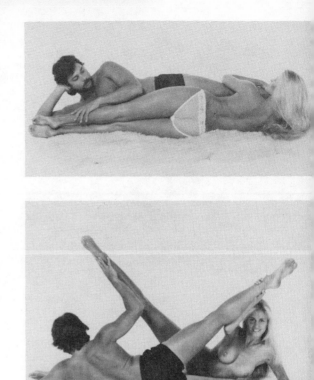

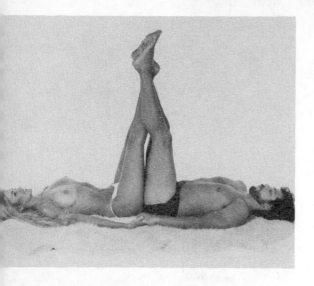

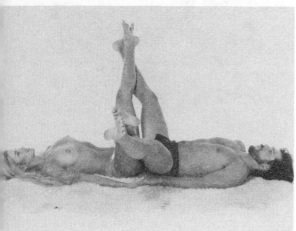

VERTICAL SPREAD

Both of you lie on your backs on the floor, moving yourselves ass-cheeks-to-ass-cheeks. This is impossible to do, of course, if you don't extend your legs up toward the ceiling. Your legs are straight and together and extended toward the ceiling, and your cheeks are touching. If you need to broaden your base of support, you can extend your arms out perpendicular to your body. Now, taking turns as one being the "pusher" and the other being the "restrainer," the pusher should keep legs together, while the restrainer should put legs outside the pusher's. The pusher should then try to open the legs, while the restrainer tries to prevent it by offering resistance. Work at it for about a minute. Then the pusher should put his or her legs outside the restrainer's and should try to close legs against resistance from the restrainer. Again, do this for about a minute, then change roles. Repeat at least five times per partner.

Benefits: Builds strength in the legs.

LEGWORK

Lie down on your back and bring one knee up to your chest. Now, have your partner kneel next to you, on the same side as the bent knee. Have him place one hand gently on your knee and the other on the heel of your foot. Now, have him gently begin exerting pressure downward on the knee and toward your head on the heel. Your lover will be able to push your leg just a bit farther than you can on your own. Do not have him push into the area of pain. You just want to loosen and stretch the muscles, taking them a matter of a half-inch or so beyond their usual limits; hold for ten seconds and gently return the leg to its neutral position. Then repeat Legwork five times, and change legs. Then change roles, with you doing it to his legs. If either or both of you are athletic, you may find your partner's legs very tight and stiff, and you may actually have to exert quite a bit of pressure to get results. But do all movements slowly and gently.

Benefits: Loosens and stretches legs.

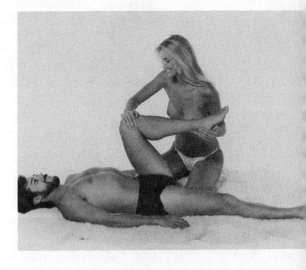

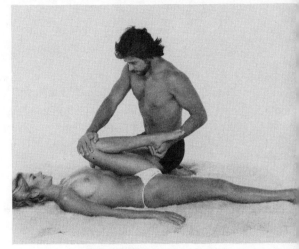

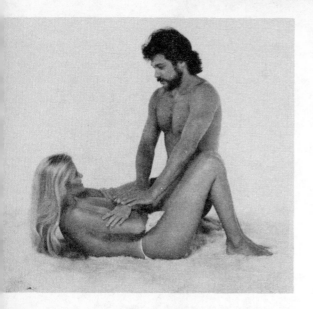

RESIST-O-SIT-UP

Lie on your back, and bring your heels up to your buttocks. Now, cross your arms over your chest as though you had died and were in your casket. Have your partner kneel next to you, close enough that with one hand he can add resistance in a downward motion against your crossed arms — not much resistance, but just enough to make it more difficult to do a sit-up. Do ten sit-ups like that, then switch roles. Now you kneel next to him and offer resistance. If your guy is really in shape, you may have to use both hands to hold him down. He may be able to do more than ten sit-ups, too. If he can, let him go at it.

Benefits: Builds abdominal muscles.

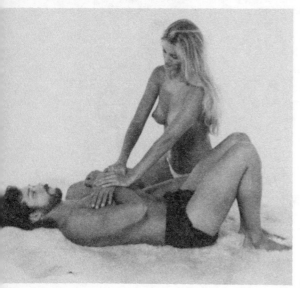

SLOW SWITCHBLADE

Lie down on your sides, face-to-face. Rest your head on your lower arm and hand, and casually drape your upper arm over your partner's waist. All work on this one comes from the legs. You can start this one. Have your lover place his upper ankle across your upper ankle. Now, as you try to raise your leg, keeping it straight all the time, he'll add a little resistance, just barely allowing you to raise it up to the highest possible point. Once it's up there, he should apply pressure to push it back down as you try to keep it up. Repeat this one five times, and then you do the same for him. When he has done it five times, reposition yourselves to do it with the legs that haven't been worked yet. Repeat five times each leg for each of you.

Benefits: Strengthens legs and hips.

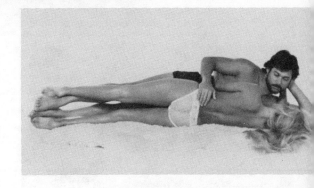

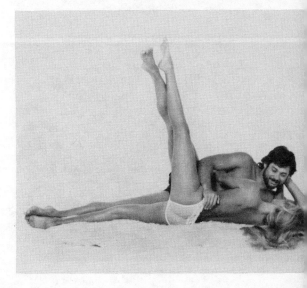

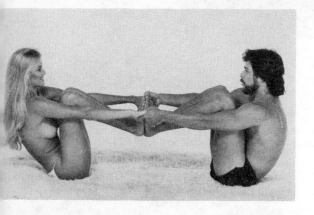

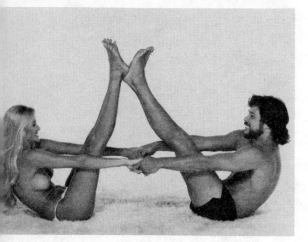

THE UPTHRUST

Sit facing each other. Join hands and, while bending knees, bring your soles against the opposite soles of your lover, so that you are balancing each other with your hands together, while your soles are together. Now, using only your buttocks as support, raise your legs, still with the soles together, until they are straight. At that point, the only portions of the soles that will be touching are the heels. Now, bring your legs back to the bent positions, with the soles in complete contact again. Then repeat the leg-straightening, but shooting for a slightly different angle, so that by the time you have ten reps of The Upthrust, you will have done almost every angle to the floor that's possible, from about 10 degrees to almost 90 degrees.

Benefits: Strengthens and stretches legs, while increasing sense of balance.

FOOT WORK

This one combines stretching and massage. Sit facing each other and extend your legs into each other's laps, keeping your legs perfectly straight. Now, each of you grasp the right leg of your partner, placing the heel in the palm of one hand to support it. Now, with the other hand, grasp the ball of the foot and slowly bend the ball of the foot toward your partner. It is essential that you both keep the leg perfectly straight. This will gently stretch the all-important Achilles tendon. Hold it for a few seconds as far as it will comfortably bend, allow it to go back to a neutral position, and then do it again. Then, still holding the foot, begin to rotate the foot so that you are loosening your partner's ankle. After you both mutually agree to stop, switch legs and repeat the process. It is usually beneficial to do each leg three times.

Benefits: Loosens tight Achilles tendons and adds flexibility to the ankle.

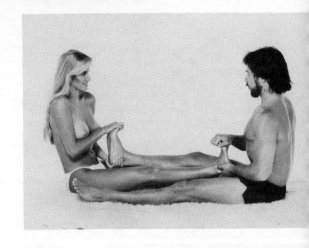

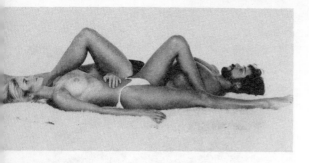

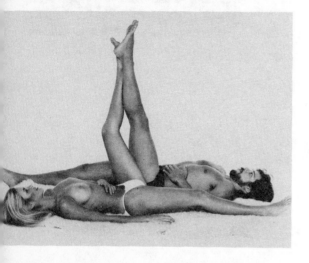

INDIAN WRESTLING

This one has a long history as a contest of strength, but we'll be using it, instead, as a method of strengthening. Both of you lie down on your backs, side-by-side, but with your heads in opposite directions, so that your left hip is against his left hip. Now, both of you raise your left legs toward the ceiling, keeping them straight, and hook your feet, just below the heel, so that if either or both of you tries to push your leg down toward the floor, you'll meet resistance from your lover trying to do the same. (In the contest version of this, the legs are brought up three times, and on the third raise, the ankles are hooked, and the contestants try to flip one another. It can be very hard on your back if done incorrectly.) Now, take turns offering resistance as the other tries to return his or her foot to the floor. Then, both of you offer an equal amount of resistance at the same time. Uncouple, and switch sides. Do each side five times.

Benefits: Strengthens the legs, and stretches the hamstring.

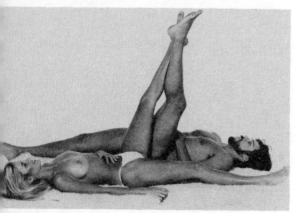

THE MOTH & THE MANTA

Have your partner lie down on his back, and have him bring the soles of his feet together. He should allow gravity to bring his knees almost down to the floor. Now, you kneel at his soles, and extend your hands to his knees. Apply very light pressure to his knees to help gravity bring his knees closer to the floor. Be very gentle in doing this; many people are very stiff and this can be very painful. Be alert for the first grimace of pain on your partner's face. Hold for five seconds, and then gently bring his knees back up, pause for a few seconds and press them down again. After ten times, reverse roles. This one is really fun when done nude, especially if the person in the role of the mantis takes his role seriously. You know what a mantis does to a moth when it catches one, don't you?

Benefits: Adds flexibility in the hips and pelvis and stretches the inner legs.

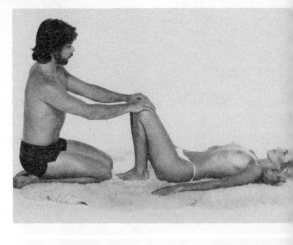

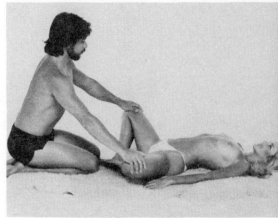

CHAPTER 7

Sexersaage

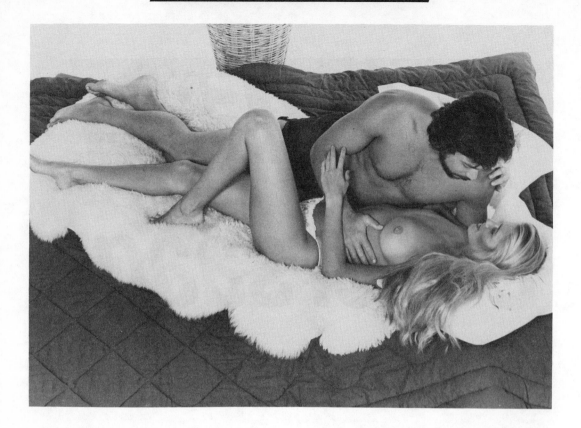

Controversy has always surrounded massage, for two reasons: First, taboos on touching among individuals vary from one culture to the next. Second, massage in the Western world has received a bad name from the term "massage parlor," a place that advertises massage but sells sex.

Before we begin our own rendezvous with a Sexersaage, I'll touch on the controversy surrounding massage.

We all know people who are cold, guarded, aloof, defensive; we also know people who are outgoing, expressive, warm, engaging. Personality, whatever form it may take, does not make a person bad or good. There are cold, defensive people who are the salt of the earth, who are scrupulously good, and there are some warm, outgoing people who would put a knife through your heart at the first opportunity.

We often stereotype people by their personalities. For example, we consider the Germans somewhat reserved, while their neighbors, the Italians, are expressive and warm. Such across-the-board statements are, however, merely generalizations.

When we pigeonhole individual families by their personalities, however, the generalizations seem to be more accurate. Consider the parents who are cold, reserved, and do not show affection for or touch each other. Usually they do not touch their children or show physical affection, either. There is a very good chance you will learn — not inherit — those same characteristics. Such coldness, aloofness and aversion to physical contact is not present in the genes; it is a learned response.

Similarly, if your parents showed their affection for each other around you, and if you perceived that they really meant it, you

ABOVE — A Sexersaage has many different applications. It can come in the wake of a heated lovemaking session, or it can lead to one. It is a way to express concern for one another: One gives totally while the other receives. TOP RIGHT — An excellent way for a woman to begin a Sexersaage session is by relaxing her man; tease him by massaging him with your hair. RIGHT — Tickling with the hair can and should be extended to all parts of the body; it can be used to set the stage for what is to come later.

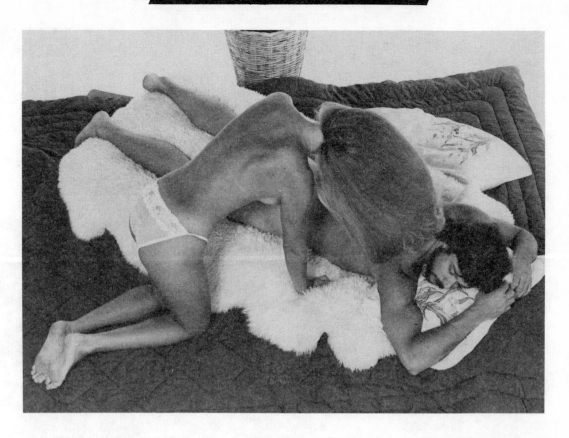

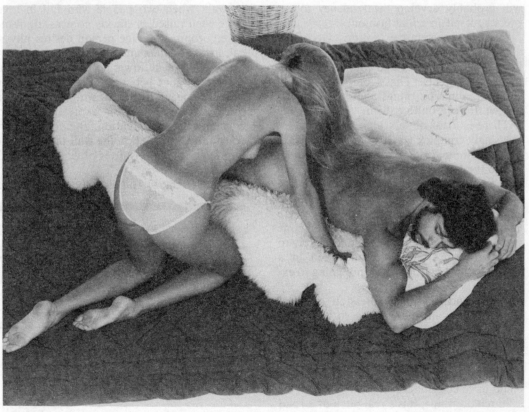

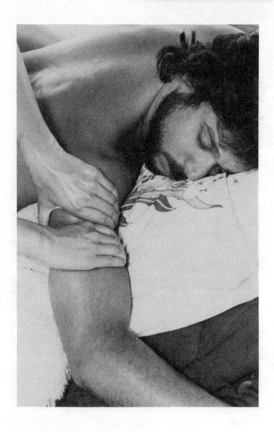

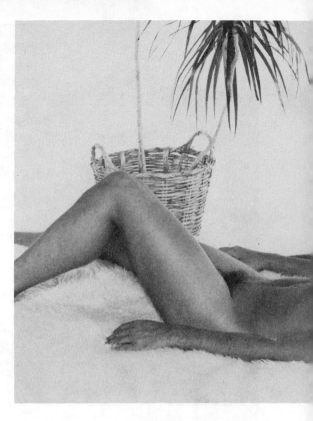

will probably develop the tendency to express yourself in a like fashion.

Of course, there are exceptions. Occasionally you will meet someone who is warm, loving, and expressive and who had two icebergs for parents. That's one of the constantly fascinating things about people: it's difficult to pigeonhole them.

There is a lot of talk about how our increasingly complex world is fostering a race of very remote, cold, analytical people; there is also the feeling that much of the touching that *is* going on today is fairly hollow and contrived. But I imagine that people are pretty much the same today as they were twenty or fifty years ago. However, someone who has been brought up "cold" is likely to have problems that a person raised in a warm, loving environment is not going to experience.

Touch and physical expression of emotions is, after all, a release, a sort of communication. If you feel restrained in expressing yourself in that way, emotions can build up inside. You might have to find other ways of expressing yourself. If you don't, you could have emotional hangups.

In relationships, it is a real bitch of a road

to walk when two people who fall in love have been raised in starkly contrasting family environments. One person desires physical, loving contact and constant communication — the way a flower needs water — while the other hides behind a fortress of ice. It can become utterly frustrating for both of them, because while the expressive person constantly seeks attention, the cold person constantly builds upon the wall that keeps it out; such a relationship is obviously headed for trouble.

It is difficult to convince the unexpressive

ABOVE LEFT — In this close-up, the proper motion that should be used on the arms and legs is clearly visible. Besides stroking toward the heart, a rubbing motion, with one hand going in one direction while the other hands goes in the opposite direction, gives best results. TOP MIDDLE — Create a pleasant atmosphere for your partner and then use liberal amounts of warm oil. TOP RIGHT — Massage the hands, but be careful not to injure delicate tendons by probing too hard. RIGHT — All strokes on the arms should be toward the heart.

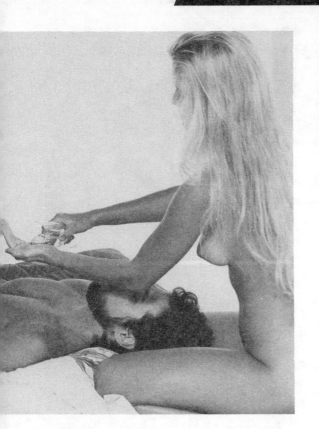

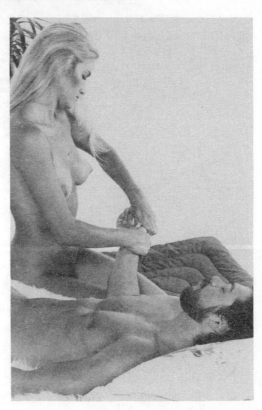

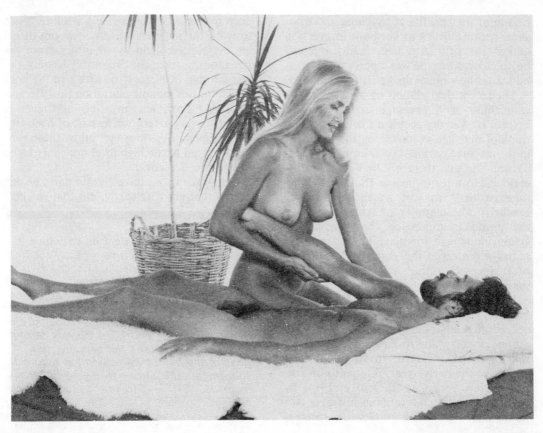

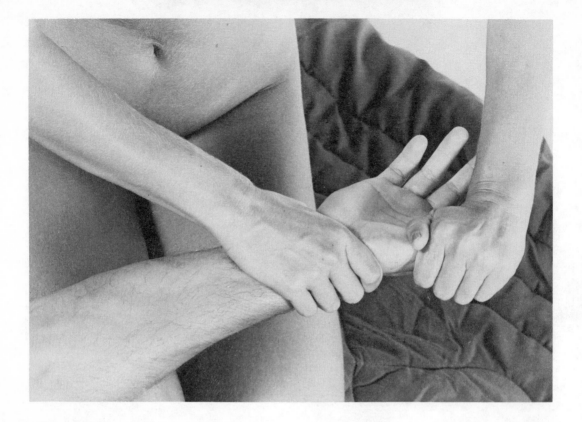

person of the benefits of touching and massage, because of his or her built-in aversion and distrust of it. And there is little one can do to change that person's perception of it, no matter how much the benefits are touted.

The recent degradation of massage by its association with massage parlors hasn't helped. How many people do you know who think of massage as something that happens in a "massage parlor," with an implied understanding that there will be sexual gratification? How many people think of "massage parlors" as just another name for brothels? The majority of Americans have the mistaken impression that massage is synonymous with foreplay. There are many *massage centers* in this country that do not offer sex, but rather a healthful, holistic massage.

If you don't care for massage, that's fine, but don't condemn it for being a ploy for sex, because it has many other benefits. Marathon runners Alberto Salazar and Waldemar Cierpinski will testify to its value. Salazar broke the twelve-year-old marathon record at New York City in October 1981, by running 26 miles, 385 yards in just over two hours and eight minutes. Salazar receives

deep massage at least twice a week in order to work the stiffness and soreness out of his leg muscles, to help avoid injury from his strenuous workouts. Cierpinski is only the second man in history to twice win the gold medal in the Olympic marathon (in 1976 and 1980). An East German, Cierpinski receives massage every afternoon as part of his training regimen. The massages allow these runners to train at the high level necessary to be the best in the world.

Let's face it, we have certain parts of our bodies that get stiff (okay, cut that snicker-

ABOVE — *When you work on your lover's fingers, pull them; do it very gently the first time. Using oil lessens the chance of pulling too hard on your partner's fingers. Massage each digit in sequence; doing the unexpected might arouse your partner, and such movements negate the purpose of the Sexersaage. TOP RIGHT — Be very careful that you do not injure the sensitive portions of the hand by pressing too hard with your fingernails; stroke with your fingertips instead. RIGHT — Stroke the stomach in circles.*

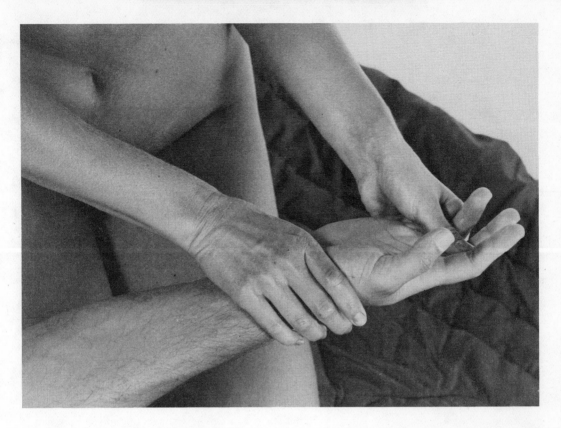

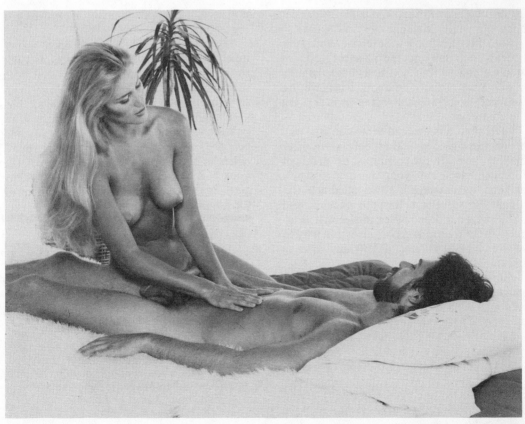

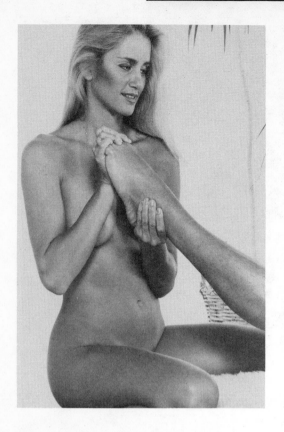

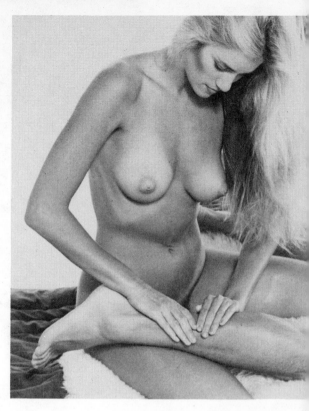

ing out there) and that could use a little relief once in a while. Massage can do the trick.

But since this book is Sexercise, and since it deals with sex and the physical you, we aren't going to lead you to believe that the massage we are talking about when we use the term Sexersaage is divorced from sex. On the contrary.

I feel that massage can be a beautiful way of expressing love, either before *or after* making love. It can certainly be excellent foreplay, arousing your partner to new heights; but massage is a two-sided activity: it can also serve to relax your partner, and put him into a deep, peaceful sleep. It is especially fitting to Sexercise, also, as a way to relieve aches, pains and stiffness after a strenuous exercise session.

So let's get right into Sexersaage. But instead of dealing with it as a foreplay to sex, let's approach it as a relaxer technique and as a tactile love exchange once the lovemaking is finished. Sit back, relax, let the tenseness drain from your body.

Although a Sexersaage is a shared experience, you must go into it realizing that it is a situation where one person is totally giving and the other is totally receiving. As love

partners, it is hoped you will take turns giving and taking.

Sexersaage should be given in a warm, quiet room and with no distractions. The room should be warm enough so that both of you are comfortable without having to resort to clothing. If a fireplace is available, you might make use of it; its warm glow serves to heighten the feeling of serenity and peace. If there is a telephone in the room, either unplug it or take the receiver off the hook and smother it with a pillow. Once begun, Sexersaage should not be interrupted for anything.

TOP LEFT & RIGHT — When you get to your lover's feet, raise them gently in your hands, being careful not to disturb him. Supporting the foot at the heel, rotate the foot slowly and carefully so that the ankle gets a good workout for flexibility. TOP CENTER — After you roll your lover over, pick up where you left off at the feet, and work on up the legs. Pay special attention to the Achilles tendon, which, in active people, gets a real workout during the day. RIGHT — Be creative with your strokes, but keep them gentle and caressing.

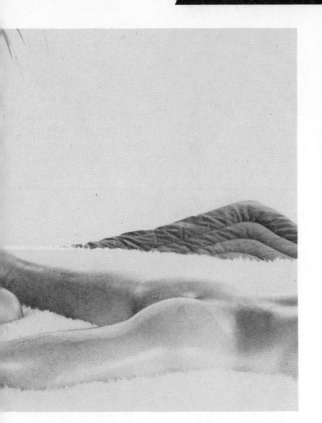

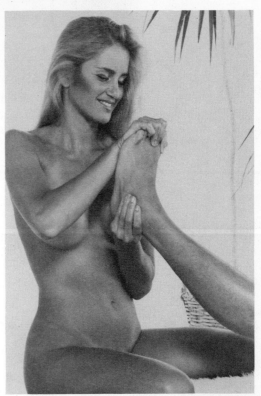

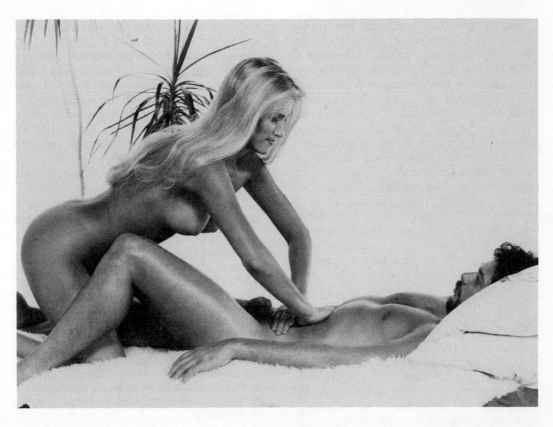

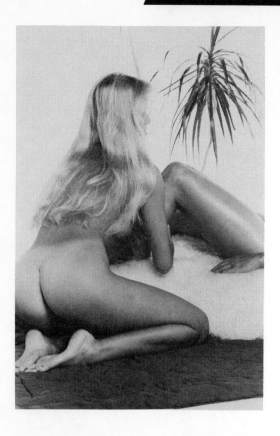

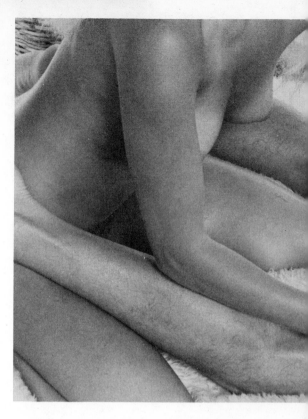

Sexersaage should be administered on the floor. First, place a pad of some sort on the floor. This is to give proper cushioning to your lover so that he remains comfortable throughout. A sleeping bag or a foam mat, or both together, will work. Now, spread a sheet over your cushioning. The sheet will absorb the massage oil. Massage oil reduces friction and increases the tactile sensations.

A massage oil needn't be anything exotic. Johnson & Johnson baby oil, or the like, works just fine. Or, you can purchase some massage oils with fragrant scents. Many of these oils are vegetable-based. You should warm the oil so that when it is applied to the body it comes as a warm, soothing balm. Cold oil will feel clammy to your partner. You can heat a small pan of water on the stove and place the container of oil in it. Keep the oil near you so that you do not have to break contact with your partner once you begin. Make sure that your hands are clean.

Now that everything is prepared, tenderly lead your partner to the mat. Your partner should lie face-up, arms at sides. Move to your partner's head, and kneel above it. Lean over and give your partner a light, butterfly's-wing-of-a-kiss on the lips, lean

back, put some oil into the palm of one hand and spread it around with the fingers of the opposite hand. From the moment that you touch your partner, you should keep physical contact during the massage. If this is your first massage, do not become apprehensive; your emotions are readily transferred through your hands. This entire experience should be a soothing one for both of you.

Start with the forehead; simultaneously make two small circles on the forehead, above the eyes. Your touch should be gentle

TOP LEFT — The Achilles tendon and calf can be massaged either from below or when your lover is on his stomach. TOP CENTER — Take your time with the hamstrings. Use liberal amounts of oil because the back of the upper leg is a large area to cover. Be careful not to press into the flesh with your fingernails. TOP RIGHT — Be sure to remember that all movements on the legs should be made in the direction of the heart. This assists the body in ridding itself of waste products. RIGHT — One of my favorite areas is the buttocks.

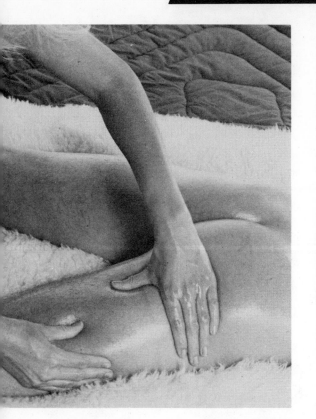

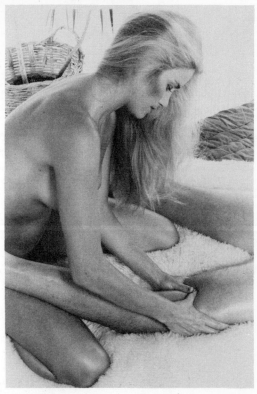

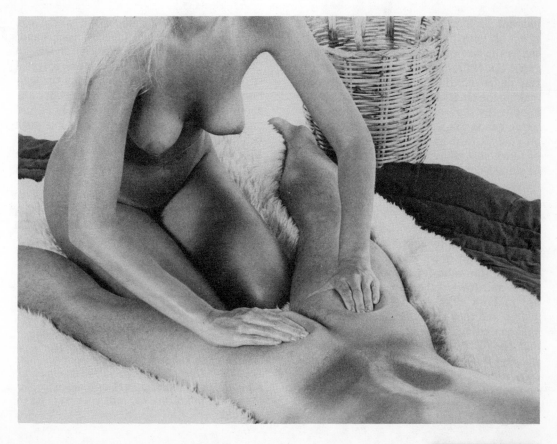

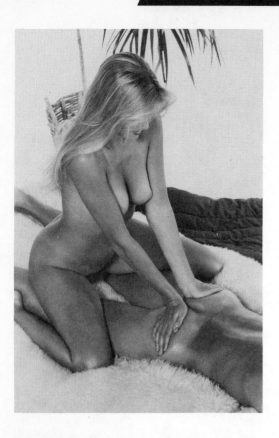

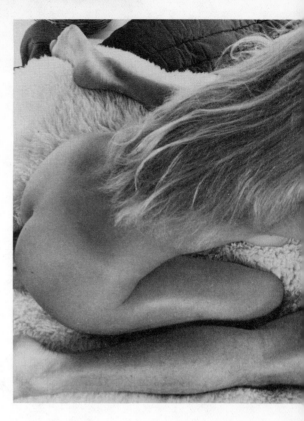

but not so light that you are having little effect on your partner's skin. Gradually increase the size of the circles, until you have swept the entire forehead. If you wish, you can linger on the forehead, progressively making the circles larger and smaller, searching out any signs of tension that your ministering hands can wash away. Your partner's only job is to relax and enjoy the sensation of touch as it takes away tension and worry; he should not be anticipating what your next move will be. You may decide to linger on the forehead for a while, to develop your technique.

Now, slide your fingers to your partner's temples, and gently massage there in small circles, sliding down to the cheeks, where you can run your fingers along the cheekbones and toward the nose; run the fingers up on both sides of the nose, massaging gently, and then gently circle the eyes. More experienced masseuses can include a light massage of the eyelids (if the partner is not wearing contact lenses), but if you are a novice, don't do it; the eyes are very delicate and your touch must be just right.

Slide the fingers back to the nose, massaging it gently, and then slide along the cheeks,

working down to the upper lip, where you can massage with one finger of each hand; circle the mouth gently. Work your way to the jaw, where you can use more forceful strokes. Work your way back along the jawbone and go to the ears. You can work the ears between the fingers; trace the lines and crevices of the ear, and gently massage behind the ear and the lobes.

From the ears, move to the neck, where you can gently roll the head as you run both hands under the neck. If your partner is relaxed, this should be extremely easy to do. If it is difficult, spend additional time on the

TOP LEFT — You can massage the buttocks any number of ways. You can work hard on them, because they are extremely fleshy and they absorb kneading very well. TOP CENTER — Run your hands directly from the backs of the legs and up onto the buttocks for best results. TOP RIGHT — This is one area where you can afford to be vigorous. Knead your lover's "cheeks" as though they were dough. RIGHT — One of the most effective manipulations is making fists and digging them into the buttocks; turn your fists as you dig.

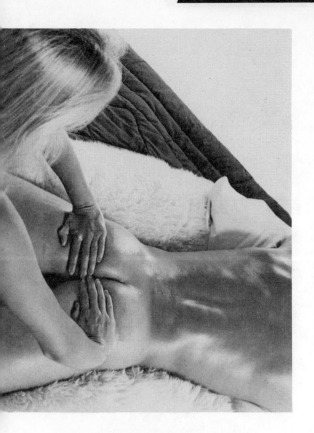
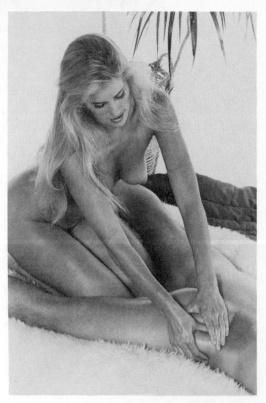
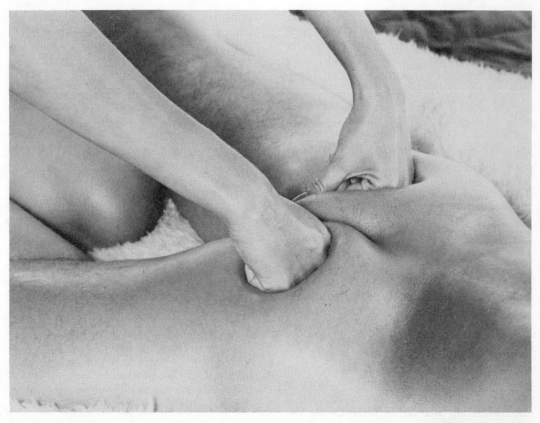

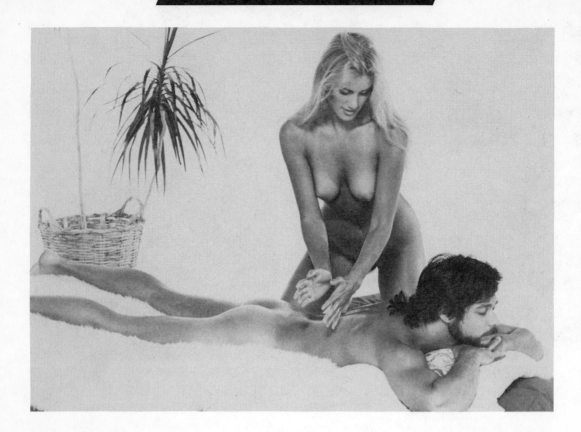

neck, helping your partner break loose some of the tension in the neck. One of the largest areas of considerable tension and stress is the shoulders. Concentrate on the neck, using your palms and fingers, but not your fingertips, which can dig into the flesh.

With one hand still caressing the neck, shift your position from behind your partner's head — gently and quietly — to your partner's side, so that you can begin working on an arm. Bring your oil with you, because you'll need to apply more oil at this point. Apply some oil directly onto the shoulder, while maintaining contact with your partner's neck. When the oil is applied, run your fingers from the neck, down through the oil, spreading it on the upper arm as you go. You can caress the upper arm as you work your way down to the wrist, making sure to maintain contact at all times.

On the arms and legs, you can massage in both directions in order to soothe the muscles, but you should use a much more forceful motion when moving toward the heart. Stroking toward the heart assists venous blood flow. The veins are closer to the skin than the arteries, consequently it is the veins that massage affects most. The veins transport waste products from the muscles back to the heart, where they can be disposed of. So when relaxing muscles you are also assisting in the elimination of waste products; this refreshes the muscles.

You can use your thumbs and fingers on the arm, and you can apply a good deal of pressure without causing discomfort to your partner. Just be sure that there is sufficient oil to lubricate your partner's skin, especially if he is hairy.

Work the arm with long, firm strokes toward the heart, and gentle — almost caressing — strokes coming down. Linger near

ABOVE — You've probably seen movies in which the fighter's trainer works him over by using a chopping motion with his hands. If you want to do it, you certainly can, but it is not necessarily something that will relax your lover; it can be quite jarring. TOP RIGHT & RIGHT — The small of the back is an area where almost everyone has soreness at some point in his life. Massage toward the spine, being very careful not to dig your fingernails into the flesh. Use the palms of your hands to exert the most pressure. Don't spare the oil.

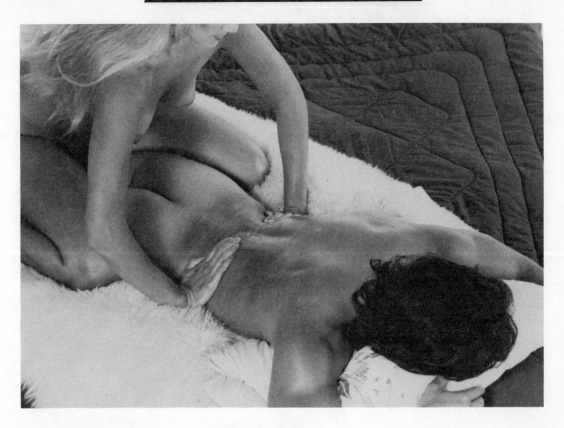

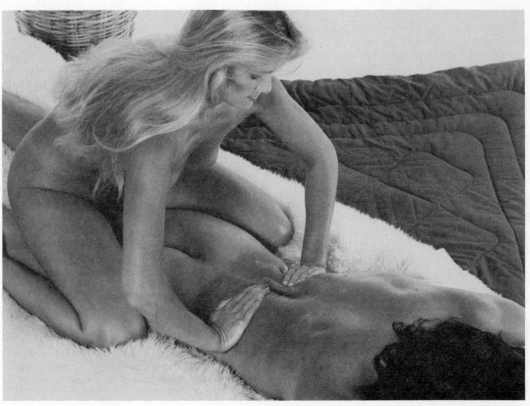

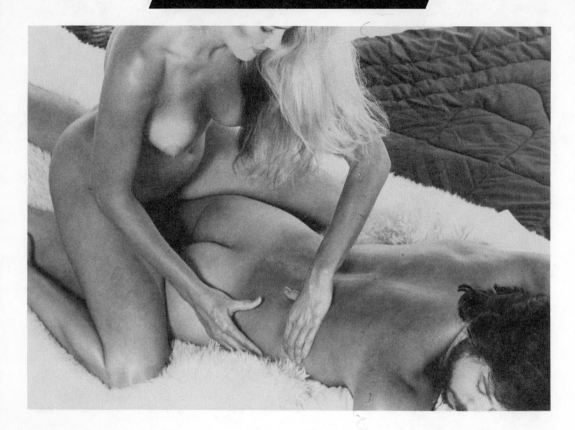

the biceps, working them over with the palms of your hands, one palm on each. Try placing your partner's forearm in your lap; by raising the upper arm off the mat, you can vibrate the large muscles of the upper arm by placing your hands on either side of the muscles. Vibration, although it seems somewhat violent when compared to the stroking you've done, is actually very relaxing for your partner.

You'll be able to tell when your efforts are having the desired results; your partner's arm becomes limp and you can move it about with ease. When you are satisfied that the arm is relaxed, move to the hand.

Take your partner's hand into yours, palm up, and knead your thumb into the palm, gently at first, and then with more force as you relax it. Knead in circular motions, using less pressure as you work near the base of the fingers.

Now, starting at the base of the small finger, pull it toward you, moving up the finger in a corkscrew motion. When you've finished all the fingers, gently press your thumb up between the fingers, running your thumb along the area between the bones and into the palm.

Turn the hand over, and execute the same ministrations on the top of the hand, stroking the fingers again. You must be careful with the hand be firm and sure in your movements, but do not dig too hard into the areas between the bones. The tendons that work the hand are, in many cases, delicate; although good effects are achieved by being firm, too much pressure could cause bruises or injury. When you have finished with the hand, rest it between your hands and warm it for a moment. Move to the other arm now. When both arms have been done, again slide

ABOVE — When dealing with the sides, maintain a firm, authoritative touch; if you lighten it, you might tickle your partner, and that will disturb his relaxed mood. TOP CENTER & TOP RIGHT — If your lover's back is firm and solid, you can knead a bit against the back of the ribs, alternating with gentle strokes from the fingers. RIGHT — Do not be afraid to sit on your lover's buttocks; they can take the pressure. From that position, run your fingers (gently) up along the spine, being very careful not to dig into the skin.

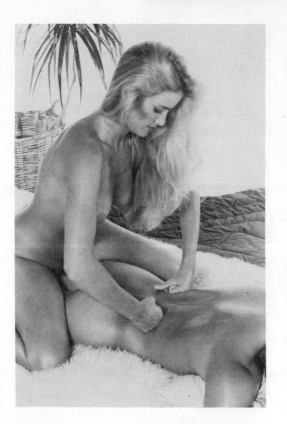

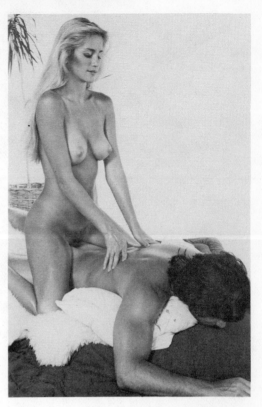

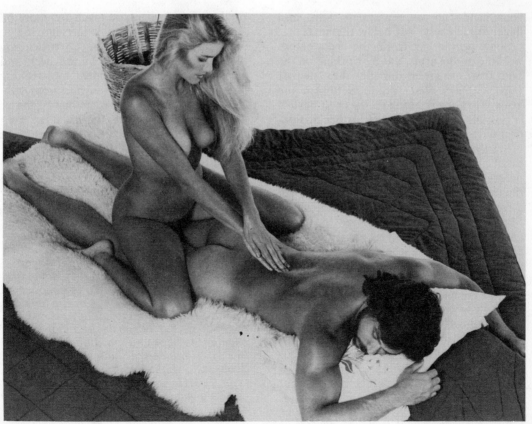

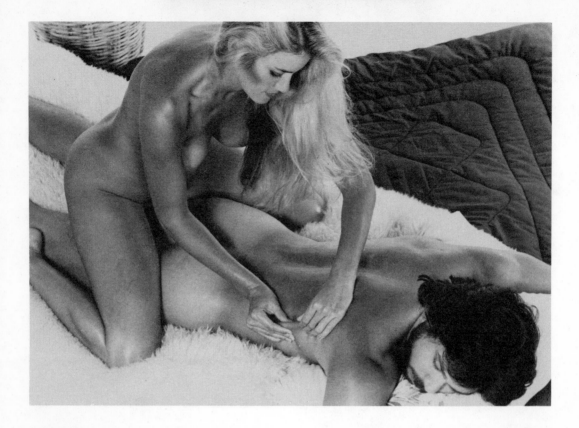

your hands up your partner's arm, and linger at the chest, just below the neck.

Some people like to do the chest before working on the arms, but by working on the arms first, you are encouraging the system of veins to carry waste products toward the heart. Then, by working on the chest next, it is possible to encourage the further dissipation of those waste products.

Start your massage on the chest by making small circles above the pectoral nearest you, progressively enlarging the circles, and using the tips of your fingers. You will quickly get a feel for how firm you should be pressing. Muscle tone varies from person to person and, as a result, you will encounter differing degrees of resistance from the person's flesh. The more toned the person is, the more pressure you can apply. Be liberal with the oil, because the chest is a very large area to cover, and you don't want to create discomfort from friction. The object is to keep the massage a uniformly pleasant experience.

You can improvise on the chest. Since it is such a large surface area, you can work it with your fingers, your palms, or with your entire hand. You should keep your hands moving constantly; to stop is to lose the

rhythm. Even when you reach for more oil with one hand, keep the other moving to maintain the rhythm. For a particularly pleasant sensation, begin at the neck and work toward the abdomen by stroking across the chest, pulling toward your own chest, constantly alternating hands; move perhaps an inch down the chest at each stroke. When you reach the abdomen, you can reverse directions.

You'll want to do both sides of the chest, so you may want to change to the other side of your lover's body to do the far side. Try

ABOVE — You can play with specific areas of flesh by gently pulling the skin up and massaging it gently between your fingers. Do not attempt this, however, on areas of the body where there is little or no loose skin. TOP CENTER — Much of the tension we pick up during a typical day resides in the shoulders. Pay special attention to the back of the neck and the shoulders. TOP RIGHT — You can give the shoulders a good, solid workout without hurting your lover. RIGHT — Some detailed attention can be given to the ear and the earlobes.

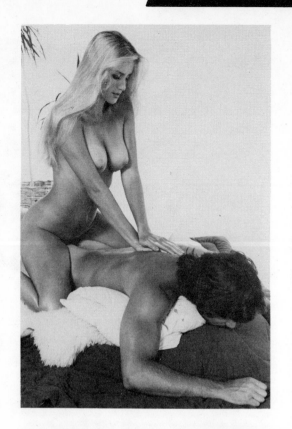

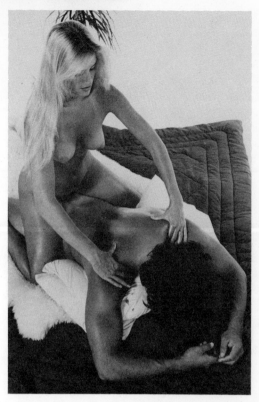

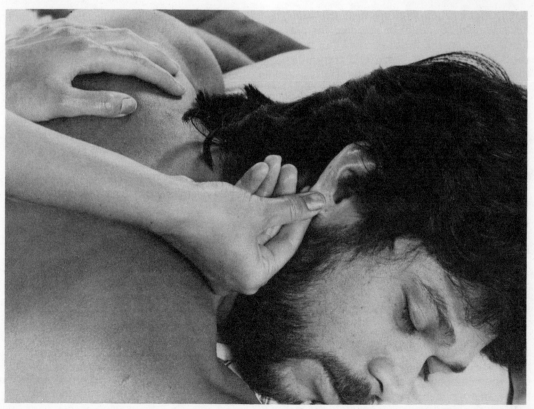

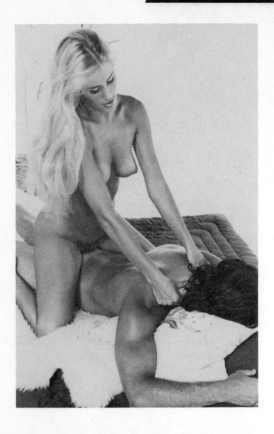

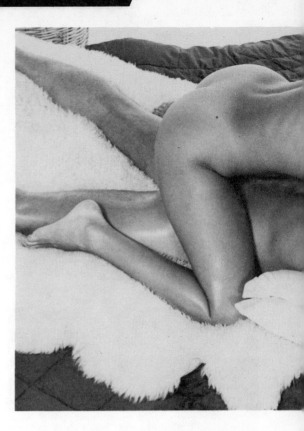

not to tickle when working near the sides, because tickling should be reserved for play before or after the massage. Tickling interrupts the feelings of peace and tranquility that you are attempting to foster.

When you are finished with the chest, move to the abdomen. Once again, begin with small circles, using the fingertips to do the massage, being careful not to dig into the flesh. Your motion should be clockwise on the abdomen, in order to move in concert with the internal organs. As with the muscle tone of the chest, it varies between individuals in the stomach muscles. If your lover is in good shape, the muscles may be somewhat taut, but as you work on them, they will likely relax. Even when relaxed, however, they will be smooth and firm; if so, you can press a bit more aggressively than if your lover's skin was somewhat slack.

You aren't going to "massage" the genitals next. Save all that. It will interrupt the relaxed, flaccid state you're attempting to achieve for your lover. There's plenty of time to deal with the genitals later; remember, you've unplugged the phone and you're both alone for the duration.

Work the hips before moving down to the legs. Linger on the hips, kneading them gently, being careful not to press too hard, as the skin between the abdomen and the legs, at least in a reclining position, is very sensitive.

Give the legs plenty of oil, because they have the most hair. Also, give them plenty of massage. The legs are your primary means of locomotion and, if your lover is active, they get an extreme amount of exertion from exercising. Even legs as tight as steel bands can be relaxed by massaging them just right.

Your massage of the legs can be more firm and vigorous than any other part of the

TOP LEFT — Pay special attention to those knots of tension in the shoulders. TOP CENTER — When you are finished with the shoulders, you can massage the arms; rub them toward the heart. TOP RIGHT — A little scalp massage goes a long way, too, so don't overlook it. NEAR RIGHT — Now comes the good part; you gave, now receive! Your lover can begin by gently massaging the forehead with his thumbs. FAR RIGHT — The massage should be gently extended over the entire face, including the cheeks and jawbone.

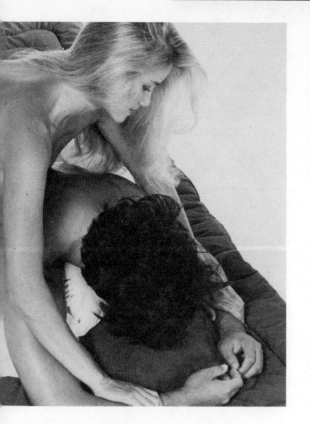

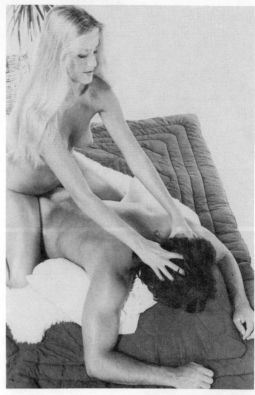

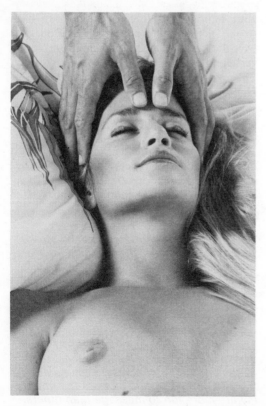

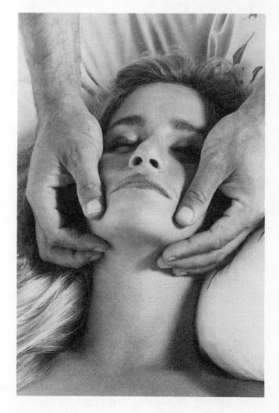

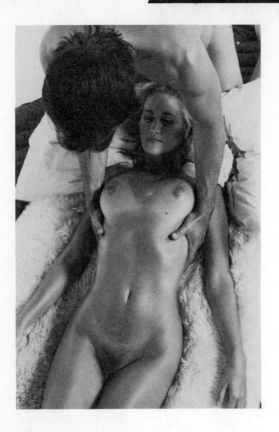
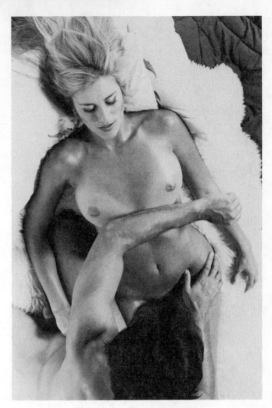

body. Because they are used so much each day, even abused, legs require more vigorous massaging to get results.

Move your hands lightly down the legs to the ankles. As with the arms, the legs should be stroked firmly, hands moving toward the heart, and gently away from the heart. Although the legs require a firm approach, be careful with the knee. The knee is a very complex joint with many ligaments and tendons. As you work on the legs, always be sure to massage the knee very, very lightly and gently.

There are several movements you can make on the legs. The basic stroke calls for pressing and driving up the leg. This should be the first stroke used. It moves wastes out of the legs and begins the relaxing process. For the next massage, work from beside the leg. Start at the top of the thigh, placing your hands across the leg, and next to each other. Now, taking a firm grip on the flesh of the leg, move your right hand forward, while you bring your left hand back; when each hand has moved about six inches, stop and reverse. This back-and-forth motion will break up any remaining tenseness or tightness in the leg. While you are doing this, ease

your hands down the leg slightly on each stroke. Remember to ease up as you pass over the knee. When you reach the ankle, reverse and begin working your way up the leg. This process has an incredibly relaxing effect!

Once you have relaxed the leg, you can caress and stroke it gently, which further relaxes it.

If you wish to work on the knee, it is best to bend your lover's leg, bringing the knee up, so that the tendons are taut instead of relaxed; there'll be less chance of injury. It is

TOP LEFT — Your lover can gently stroke your sides from a position behind your head; he should gently "lift" your torso while stroking. ABOVE — The forearm can be used as an effective massage tool, especially on large surfaces such as the chest and back. TOP RIGHT — A little reminder that your lover is still awake can keep things interesting. NEAR LEFT — Strokes to the arms should be repeated, gently and in the direction of the heart. FAR RIGHT — Certain parts of the anatomy are more fun to massage than others.

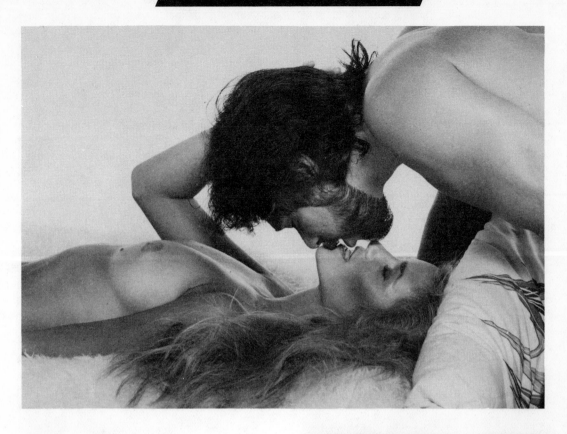

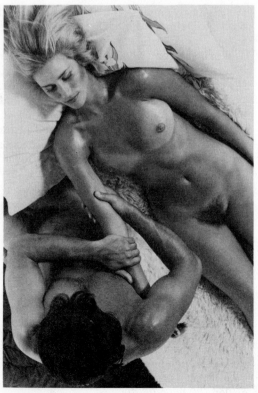

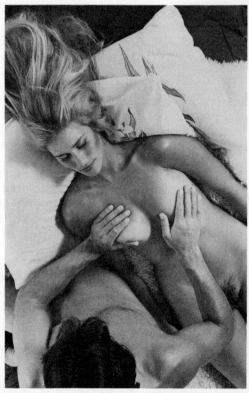

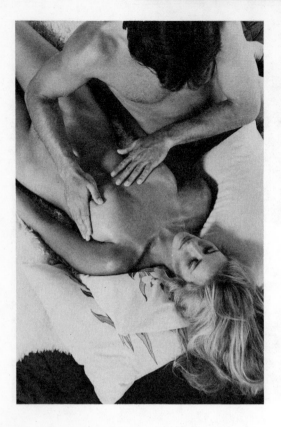

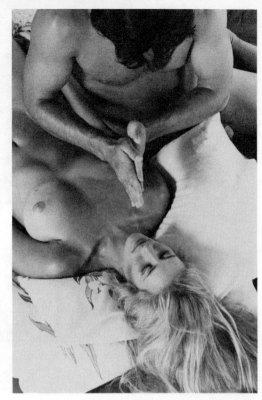

best to use the heel of your hand in massaging the knee, to lessen the chance of poking a finger into a sensitive spot. When you are finished, return the leg to a straight position, and move to the feet.

Cultures of the Orient place a great deal of importance on the feet, feeling that they are a central point of the body. Feet are very important in acupressure and acupuncture. If your lover is a runner, there are other reasons why the feet are important. I have a friend who, the night before a marathon, in addition to having his carbohydrate-feed, has an hour foot massage from his lover. It prepares him for the next day, and usually puts him to sleep on a night when — for some — it is difficult to fall asleep.

Most people are quite ticklish in their feet and, as I mentioned before, the massage is to relax a lover, not to rouse him. When working on the soles, use a clenched fist to massage. Using a fingertip is more likely to elicit a tickling reaction because of its small surface area. The foot can be held at the heel with one hand, while with your other fist, you firmly knead the sole. You needn't worry about injuring the bottom of the foot. The top of the foot, however, is another sto-

ry. It's fairly fragile, so it should be stroked with the palm of the hand, rather than the fist.

Work the foot while you have it in your hands — turning and twisting it at the ankle. If your massage has been successful to this point, the foot should be very relaxed and move freely. When flexing or twisting it, push it to the point of resistance, and just a bit beyond. The twists and turns you execute on the foot will be refreshing for your lover. The moves are made possible without injury because the foot is not bearing weight.

TOP LEFT — The breasts can be massaged, gently, using a fondling, circular technique. ABOVE — You can use the chopping motion on the area above the breasts, but do be gentle. TOP RIGHT — Massage the stomach in a circular, smooth motion, and exert pressure from the palm, not from the fingers; this way you'll avoid injuring delicate internal organs. NEAR RIGHT — Be very careful not to dig the fingers into the abdomen. FAR RIGHT — A nice touch, before moving to the legs, is to stroke the neck gently.

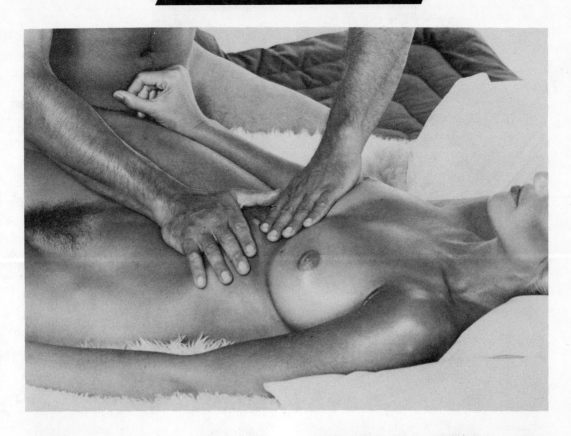

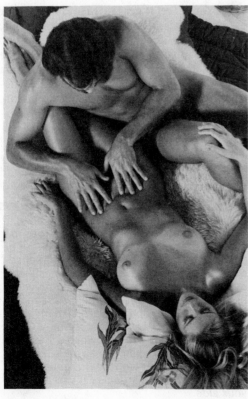

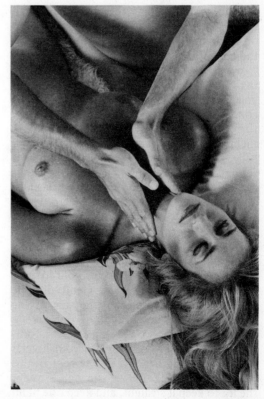

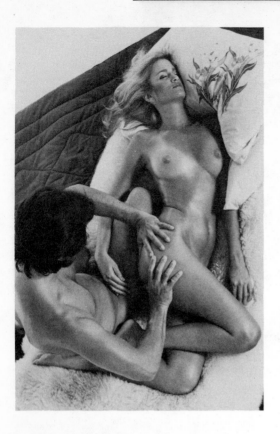

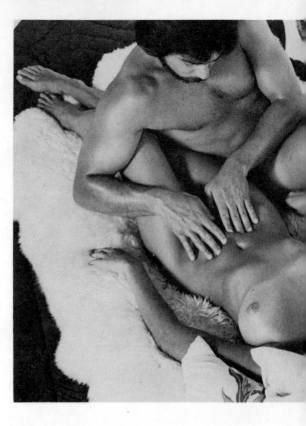

While you have the foot in hand, so to speak, rub oil into the toes and, as you did on the hand, run your finger gently between the bones that connect the foot with the toes. Now, grasp a toe in your fingers, and gently tug it away from the foot. Don't worry that you'll pull the toe off the foot; it is well connected. Tug gently at first, and then more firmly. The oil will prevent you from pulling them too hard, because they'll be so slippery. The sensation of tugging on the toes is similar to the pleasure some people get from cracking their knuckles. You may occasionally pull a toe that responds with a *popping* sound; if you've used oil on it, you don't have to worry that you've dislocated it.

When toe massage is done, I like to follow it with an Achilles tendon stretch from the toes. This is especially good for your lover if he is athletic and runs a lot. Gently lift the foot to your chest, placing the sole of the foot onto your chest, keeping your lover's leg straight. Now, slowly lean into the foot, tilting your upper body toward your lover's head so that the bending of the foot begins to cause resistance. Leave your hands under the leg to keep it straight, and keep one hand on the tendon where it joins the heel of the

foot. You'll feel it get taut. Hold it there for a few seconds, back off for five seconds, then lean into it again. Using your fingers on the hand in contact with the bottom of the Achilles tendon, begin a massaging action (not too unlike the male masturbation motion) up and down the Achilles tendon, which is just behind the ankle. This will increase blood flow to the tendon, and the tendon will give more as you put pressure on it. Alternate putting on pressure, and backing off. With each repetition, the tendon should become more flexible.

TOP LEFT — Although most massages are given to a person who is reclining either on his front or his back, some unusual sensations — and especially sensual ones — can be generated by being turned on your side so that your hips can be massaged. TOP CENTER — I particularly like my lover to linger over my abdominal region. TOP RIGHT — The hip area provides a base for some good, vigorous massage. RIGHT — Your lover will be able to get a good grip on your abdominal muscles if you are on your side.

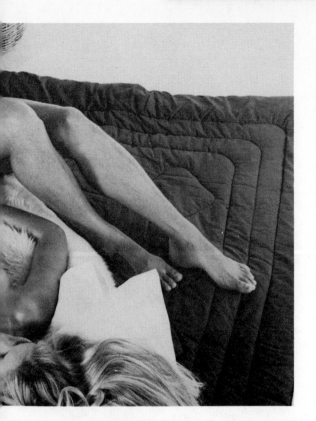

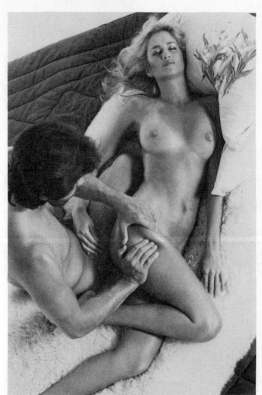

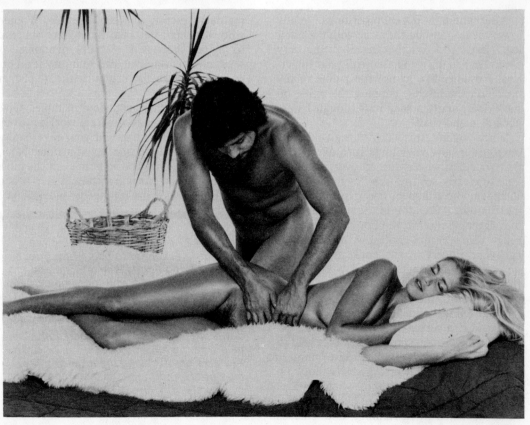

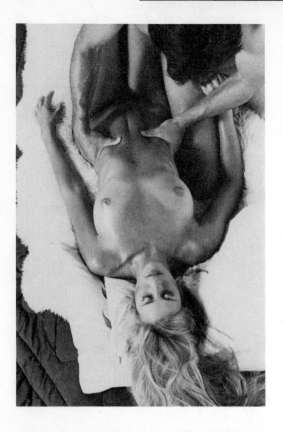
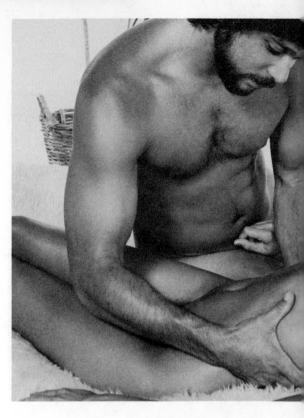

After about a dozen repetitions, gently lower the leg, and do the same with the other leg. Next, work on the ankles, being very careful not to dig into them with your fingertips. I usually like to use the palms of my hands on the ankles, cupping the ankle on both sides, and working it as though I were packing a snowball.

When you are finished with the ankle, the next step is have your lover turn over. Now that your partner has turned over, you'll be able to clearly see the Achilles tendon. For someone who is active, this is probably the most important tendon in the body; and it's the biggest tendon in the body. Remembering to keep constant contact with your lover, run your fingers to the back of the heel; now, run your fingers down a centerline from the heel to the calf, that large muscle directly below the back of the knee. The Achilles tendon attaches at the back of the heel, and it is very narrow at that point, expanding as it extends up the calf. It is held to the calf muscle by a multitude of minute connecting tissues. Running sends shock up through the Achilles tendon, when the heel strikes the ground; additionally, it is somewhat shortened when running, and it needs

regular stretching to keep it supple. Women who wear high-heels day in and day out tend to have shortened Achilles tendons. A shortened tendon can lead to injury if an exercise program is begun without proper stretching.

So what's the next step? Simple. Give those Achilles tendons a real working over. Move forward and spread your lover's legs slightly, straddling one leg at a time. Now, remembering that you want to exert the most pressure when stroking toward the heart, give the back of the leg a generous ration of

ABOVE LEFT — When massaging the sides, it is essential to use a firm grip; if you touch too lightly, you'll tickle and any tickling should be saved for foreplay, after the Sexersaage. TOP CENTER — Your lover can run his hands up or down your sides. I like him to do my sides both on the way down my body to my feet, and again when he's working his way back up. TOP RIGHT — I also enjoy having my lover grip my hips firmly and then massage them vigorously. RIGHT — I really love to have my abdomen massaged and rolled.

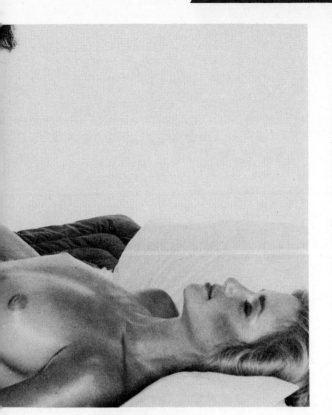

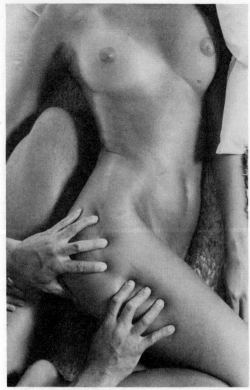

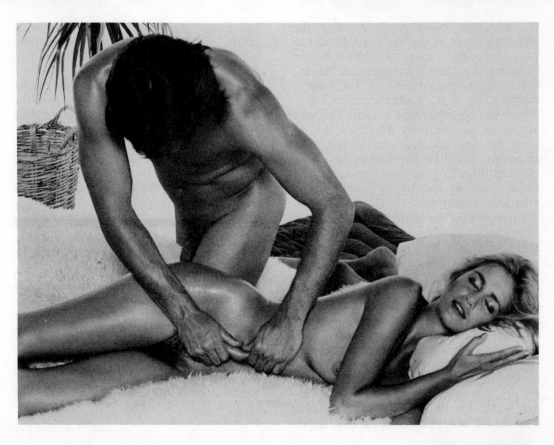

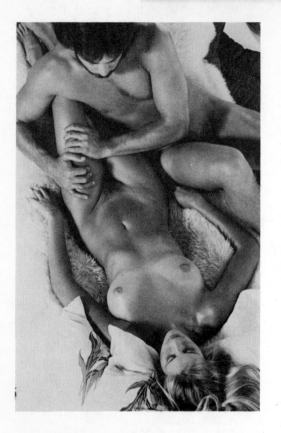

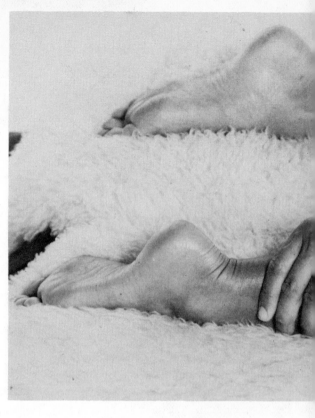

oil, and then begin *gently* stroking the Achilles tendon, all the way from the heel to the calf. I'm stressing *gently* because if your lover is active, there is a chance that the tendon is slightly bruised and sore. You want to warm it up first, gradually loosening it before you begin working it hard. This way you avoid causing pain. You'll be able to sense tightness and soreness through your fingertips. You'll be surprised by what you can feel through your fingertips once you begin practicing and tuning yourself in to your lover's body.

Keep working the tendon until you feel it soften from becoming relaxed. As it softens, begin working it with the fingertips, being careful never to dig into the flesh; digging in with the fingers can cause tears and bruises.

Now, move to the calf. The calf has closely packed muscle fibers, and is one of the most worked muscles in the body (the heart gets the most work). It tends to stiffen up fairly easily during exercise, and can stay that way for a long time afterward. It is an easy muscle to work on, however. It is large, smooth, and all the fibers run in one direction (parallel to the body). As with the tendon, the calf may be quite sore and stiff, and

you should start your workout on it very gently, with a stroking motion rather than jumping right in there and kneading it to death.

Use the palms of your hands, and remember to stroke a little more firmly *toward* the heart, merely sliding the palms over the flesh on the way back toward the foot.

As the calf fully relaxes, you can do what you did with the biceps; put your hands on the sides of the muscle and vibrate it rapidly. Vibration loosens the muscle and more fully relaxes it.

TOP LEFT — I enjoy a massage with as much physical contact from my lover as is humanly possible. I get a kick out of having him lean against me while he is working on one or another part of my body. TOP CENTER — The Achilles tendons along the back of the leg can be very tender and sore if you run or exercise a lot; it is an especially good place to get a massage. TOP RIGHT — The bottom of the foot is very sensitive and must be massaged forcefully to avoid tickling; do not press too hard with the fingers or thumbs.

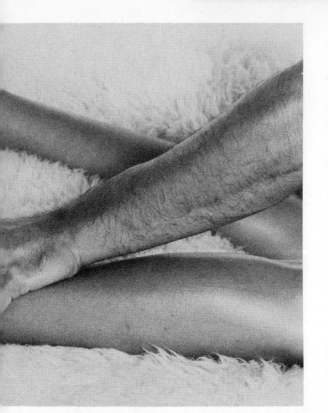

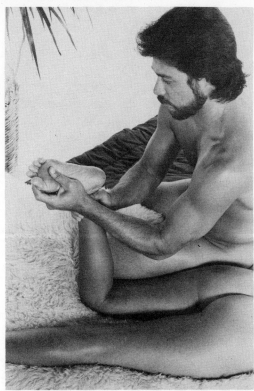

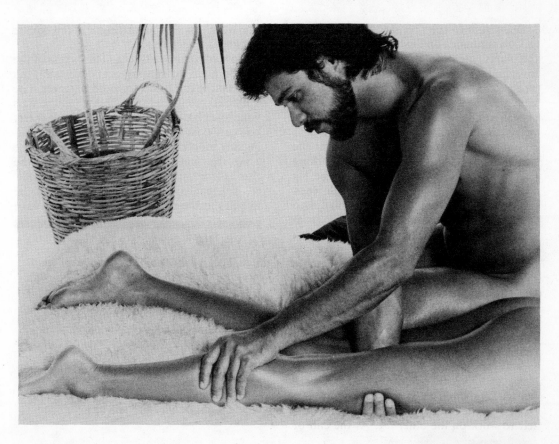

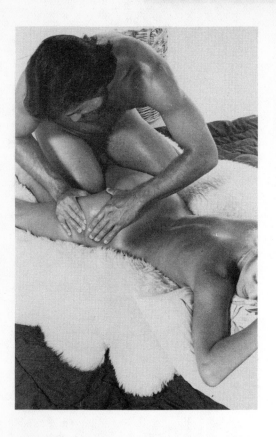

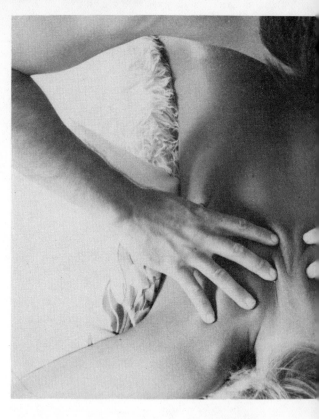

Being sure to keep contact with the body, move your hands up the back of the thigh — the hamstring. Move to the side of your lover, or else straddle the leg. Be careful when moving your hands from the calf to the hamstring. You don't want to put too much pressure on the back of the knee, as this is a very sensitive and easily damaged area.

Spread a generous amount of oil over the hamstring area, and you will begin working it from just above the knee. Grasp the leg with both hands — the hands beside each other — and then, similar to what you did on the upper arms, roll one hand away from you (if you are kneeling beside your lover) and the other one toward you. Alternate twists, as though you were screwing together the ends of two pipes. With each movement, slide your hands an inch or so farther up the leg until you reach the buttocks; at that point, reverse the process, stroking more than twisting. Stroke more firmly toward the heart.

This can be done for as long as it takes to break up any remaining tension in the hamstring. When one leg is finished, slide your hand over the buttocks and reposition yourself to work on the other leg. At the end of

the work on the hamstrings, a few gentle strokes is a nice touch.

Now come the buttocks. This is one of the easiest areas to massage, and certainly an area that is fun to do for both partners. The buttocks are extremely fleshy, and unless your lover has recently pulled a muscle there, you can work them vigorously without causing any problems; it is most pleasurable. Use a vigorous kneading technique, working the cheeks from one side and then from the other. You can also get good response to the muscles in the buttocks by doing this: make

TOP LEFT — As much as I love to massage my lover's buttocks, I love even more to have him massage mine. A firm, kneading movement works wonders to make the muscles more supple. TOP CENTER — The shoulders are the receptors of most of the day's tensions, so take plenty of time to work that tension out. Use vigorous strokes and plenty of oil. TOP RIGHT — The upper arms should also be stroked tenderly and often. RIGHT — The buttocks should be kneaded as you apply your weight behind the arms.

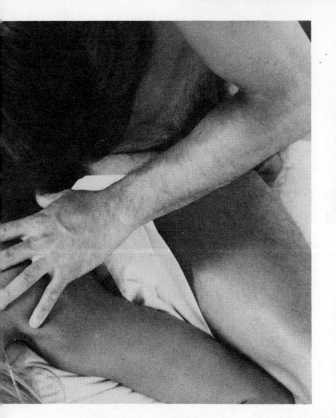

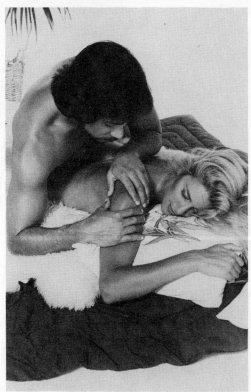

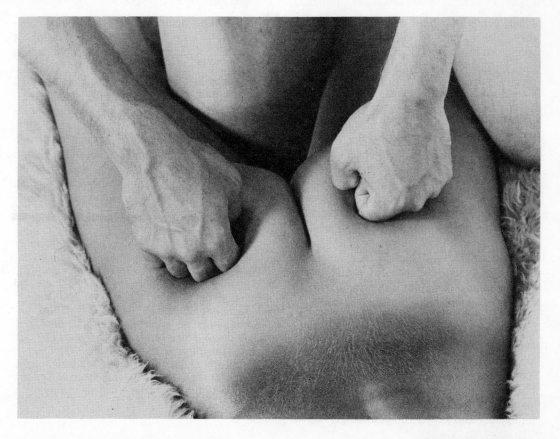

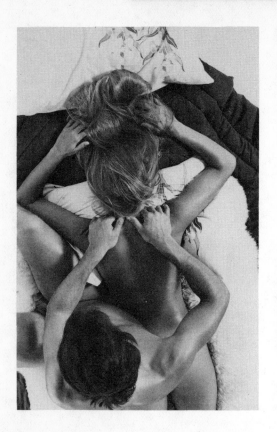

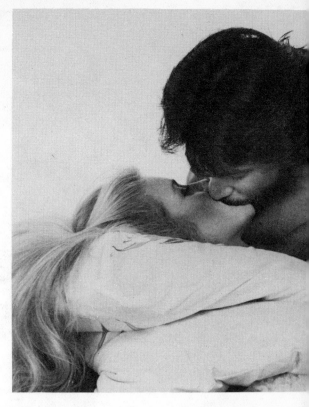

a fist, gently placing it on the buttocks and, then, use a turning motion, applying pressure from the arm with your body weight behind it. Keep moving the fist around the buttocks as you're doing this. Save any sexual teasing you might consider here until your are completely finished with the massage. You've still got the most important part to massage.

The back is a huge area to cover and, as a result, you should break it down into segments. As you know, the spine runs vertically up the back and is the connection between the hips and the head. Inside it, like conduits of the ancient Roman water system, rest all the nerves that control the movements of your entire body. All signals from the brain to the body travel down the spine, nerve pathways branching out along the way. The spine is an extremely important part of the body, and should be treated carefully.

Staddle your lover with your legs bent at the knee. You should be kneeling, resting on your knees and lower legs. Gently slide your hands up your lover's back, on either side of the spine. When you reach the neck, place your index fingers on either side of the spine and gently and slowly run your fingers down your lover's back, feeling each of the vertebrae as you go. Do not press too hard. It takes a real expert to know just how hard a spine can be pressed before causing injury. In your massage, just press very gently with the tip of your finger, running your fingers from the neck to the buttocks; do *not* dig into the spine.

Now, the entire back remains with its two equal halves. You can work on one side at a time with both hands, or you can work the full back, with one hand ministering to each side. This close to the end of the massage,

TOP LEFT — I also love to have my lover run his thumbs gently down along both sides of my spine. You have to be careful, however, not to dig into the skin or damage the backbone. TOP CENTER — The end of a massage, especially when it is of the Sexersaage type, can be the most pleasant part of all. The experience can lead to some terrific lovemaking. TOP RIGHT — Your body should feel energized and supple ready for love. RIGHT — Enjoy your Sexersaage, and let it lead to whatever may come.

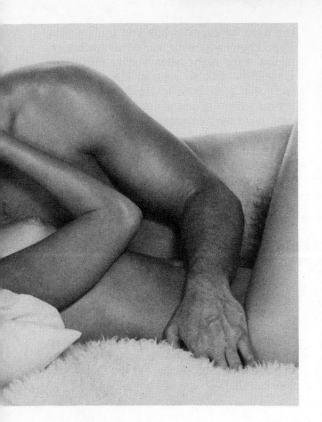

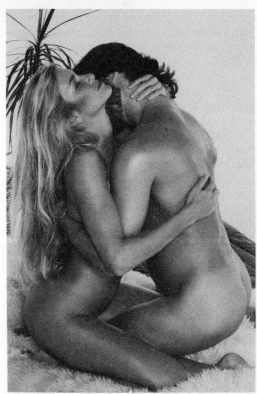

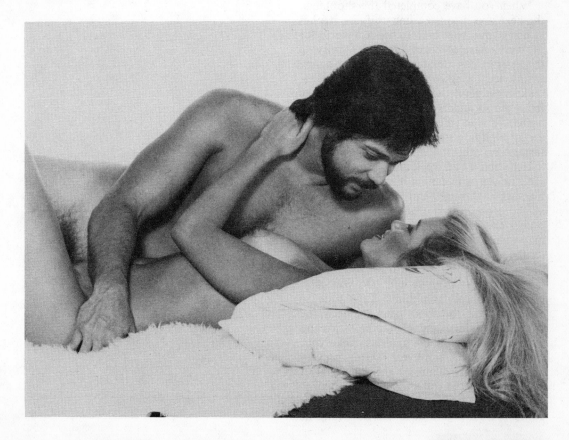

you don't want to rouse your lover with each hand going in a different direction. Synchronize your hands as they work the back.

On the back, you can use your entire hand to knead the flesh (make sure to use plenty of oil, because the back is a rather substantial area to cover properly), which allows you to cover more area with each motion. Or, you can use the tips of the fingers, but make sure you keep your palms very close to the body as you do this, so that you do not dig in with the fingertips. Work your way up the back to the shoulders using circle motions. The shoulders and the back of the neck are the depositories of many of our tensions, apprehensions, worries and problems. You may frequently find that your lover is quite stiff and tight. When you do, begin by gently stroking and rubbing your fingers held together. As the shoulder begins to loosen, grab a shoulder in your hands, kneading it gently. Work back and forth across the shoulders. The muscles, which felt like taut cables when you began, should now feel like cookie dough. Your lover will not mind if you spend some extra time on the shoulders.

When you have completed the shoulders, the next step is to use some unifying strokes to bring your lover back to the real world for the next phase of Sexersaage. The unifying strokes can best be done by kneeling beside your lover. Using your fingertips like a rake, make long, gentle, teasing strokes all the way from the shoulders, down the back, to the buttocks, into the hamstrings, and back again. Unifying strokes can be done a little faster than others.

If he had a bad week and you want to be kind to him, you can let him sleep when the massage is through. But since a massage is all giving on the part of the masseuse, and all taking on the part of the poor victim, you may want to have some fun at this point. After the unifying strokes, gently roll him over onto his back. Begin "teasing" you partner using a feather or your hair. Do you get a positive arousal from him? Take time to tease the chest, the upper arms, the neck, the sides, the insides of the thighs, the hands and feet, and ultimately the genitals. Take your time in doing this, however. Teasing is a very nice part of any relationship, and it almost invariably ends in some terrific lovemaking.

Challenge your lover to a battle of self-control. Challenge him to see how long he can keep hands off while you titillate your lover's body with your hair or the feather or, if you want to be extravagant, with a fur glove. You can also use your lips and tongue to further tease your lover; the oil that you get on your tongue isn't going to harm you (you can buy some that is flavored to taste good), and you can get some wonderful reactions with just little flicks of the tongue on the right spots. Have at it.

Sexersaage, as I stated at the beginning of this chapter, is an excellent way to rid yourself and your lover of the troubles of the outside world preparatory to enjoying each other lovingly. But it is also an excellent way to take turns completely relaxing each other *after* lovemaking. And as anyone who is in touch with the real world knows, a good session of relaxation is worth its weight in gold. And who better to give you that golden rest than your most intimate friend?

Intimacy is best preserved when you keep in touch with your feelings and the feelings of your lover, and Sexersaage is the perfect connection.

CHAPTER 8

Sexercise with Rhythm

A great proliferation of exercise classes has been set to music. There is Aerobic Dancing, Jazzercize, Jazz-Aerobics, Exergenics, Dance Aerobics, Aerobacize, and so on. You can no longer tell the program without a program.

I'm not being cynical, though. I think that they're wornderful. A concept that can get so many people out doing so much exercising is terrific. It just becomes confusing to me to keep track of which program is which. Maybe all the different programs whould unite under one banner, calling themselves something descriptive — like The Dance of Life Society.

The aerobic dance programs are built upon a very simply — but very viable — concept: keep moving in order to gain an aerobic effect. The movements are more fun and more interesting when done with a group, and they are infinitely more fun and interesting done to music; the body can get into a rhythm with the music and flow through one body movement after the other. The movements are kept continuous enough that you're out of breath, but just under the threshold of anaerobic distress. Dancing can have the same aerobic affect as running, cycling or swimming.

Sexercise with Rhythm is exactly like that — yet completely different. The dance programs rely heavily upon body movement. Our program also relies heavily upon body movement, but in an exercise mode.

Our emphasis is on muscle development and toning to a more serious degree than most aerobic dance programs. We allow for developing aerobically, among other options. Some programs are designed as warm-up body movement sequences, which are a springboard for getting in a more advanced sequence. Or they can be used as a loosening-up sequence. Some are done on a very simple level, but are designed to heighen yuor awareness of body movement and to, I'll be frank, flaunt your newfound ability at body movement and exercising.

Other programs are more advanced (taking Sexercises from all three levels); they stress you after warmup, and may have a portion or two in the middle where you back off considerably to allow your body to catch up with your enthusiasm. Others are purely sensual. And then there's the fifteen-minute White Fire sequence that you'll want to try out on your lover next time you both have a long evening together at home.

All of the sequences are created to complement the accompanying music. This music is generally available at a good record store. You're going to hear everything from rock and soul to jazz and classics, country and rhythm and blues; some music defies classification.

You don't want to have to interrupt yourself once you get started, of course, by changing records. You can get around that by taping the songs as they are outlined. Once you have the tapes, you can put them in a Sony Walkman and go through your routines wired for sound; you can set up a portable tape recorder just about anywhere and do your routine, or you can play your tape in a fidelity sound system and pretend that you're doing your routine in a concert hall.

What follows, then, are different routines for different moods, for differing lengths of time (so you have the option to fit the routine to your schedule). Put that music together and get your act in gear. Let's get down and Sexercise!

PUMPING DAISIES

A very basic routine (lasting twenty minutes, thirty-four seconds) using Sexercises from the Casual Level. Move smoothly from one exercise to the next, creating your own "bridges" between specific exercises that will unite them into a cohesive entity. Remember to base your exercising tempo on the music. Turn the music up and flow with it. The music for this session is from the film *"Chariots of Fire,"* but is one continuous piece of music. Close your eyes as you exercise, listen to the wind and the surf, and let the music carry you with it.

Artist: Vangelis
Album: Chariots of Fire
Record Company: Polydor
Album's Serial Number: PD-1-6335
Side: Two

The Sexercises

Timer	Sexercise	Remarks
00:01	Casual #1 — Head Roll	Start on your knees, rolling your head to the sound of the wind and the waves
01:46	Casual #4 — Feline Stretch	Begin as the piano comes in
03:42	Casual #5 Silk Crossover	As the waves diminish and the piano softens
05:42	Casual #9 — Long Ride	The waves return; move up and down to the rhythm of the waves and the piano
07:04	Casual #10 — Long Arch	A flurry of piano, eventually becoming dramatic; go with the music
08:39	Casual #12 — The Turtle	After the crescendo, follow the piano solo
10:20	Casual #16 — The Sphinx	Roll into the mysterios Spinx at will
11:30	Casual #17 — Sphinx Drop	The tempo and the waves build, and so do you
12:21	Casual #19 — Pelivic Punch	Bombastic music; punch to the beat
13:29	Casual #6 — Savage Cycles	The piano theme comes up strong, then drops; pace yourself and allow your leg speed to match the music
17:20	Casual #24 — Stargazer	Begin as the electronic pulses turn your body into a laser to the stars
20:15	Stand straight, head up	As the wind returns, imagine it blowing through your hair at the end of a perfect Sexercise with Rhythm routine

L.E.D. (Long, Easy Distance)

This session, which lasts for twenty-three minutes and forty-two seconds, is primarily strength-building and is very aerobic; you should work up a good sweat and you should tire in this one. You are going to do only five of the Casual Level Sexercises, but you are going to do them to near-exhaustion. If you find that you can't make it all the way through on any one of these, or on more than one, relax! You'll eventually be able to do it. These build a tremendous capacity for going long. Do the session at the same pace as the music. Once you get these five Sexercises down, you may want to substitute others; although the five are designed to work a wide range of muscle groups, you can customize it to work muscles you are particularly interested in developing.

Artist: Louis Clark
Album: Hooked on Classics
Record Company: RCA
Album's Serial Number: AFL1-4194
Side: One

The Sexercises

Timer	Sexercise	Remarks
00:01-05:02	Casual #48 — The Dog	Whip it with the beat; great for the legs and hips
5:03-11:43	Casual #41 — Leg Roll	A nice, easy pace; think romantic thoughts and let the memories flow
11:44-14:45	Casual #39 — Hippie-Hippie Shake	Let yourself really go on this one; you'll make the changeover in the middle of this cut, at the introduction of "Ride of the Valkyries"
14:46-17:50	Casual #31 — Lady Ape	Do the monkey
17:51-23:42	Casual #25 — The Sprinter	Get athletic, get on the track

FEMME FARTLEK

Fartlek is a method of training used in running; the runner changes speed frequently during the workout. The runner might key on a landmark up ahead and pick up the pace tgo that point, then back off for the next quarter-mile. It is an effective technique for learning pacing, and for throwing speedwork into a road workout. We'll do that in this session of Sexercise with Rhythm. The sequence of Sexercises is designed to warm you up with Casual Level, then lead you into Intimate and Intense, finally bringing you back down. Each Sexercise is designed to go with one song, and to be done for the song's duration. Remember to try to match the beat of the song. The three albums are by English groups: the Beatles, the Rolling Stones, and Led Zeppelin; there's old music and new music, mostly fast but some slow. I've arranged this sequence so that you'll have to change position between many of the Sexercises. Changing position is also a form of exercise within the exercise sequence; try to make the changes smoothly between songs, and be creative coming up with movements that get you smoothly from one Sexercise to the next. Go to it!

Artist: The Beatles
Album: Reel Music
Record Company: Capitol
Album's Serial Number: SV-12199
Side: One

Artist: Led Zeppelin
Album: II
Record Company: Atlantic
Album's Serial Number: SD-8236
Side: Two

Artist: The Rolling Stones
Album: Tattoo You
Record Company: Rolling Stones Records
Album's Serial Number: COC-16052
Side: One

The Sexercises

Timer	Sexercise	Remarks
00:01	A Hard Day's Night	Casual #4 — Feline Stretch
02:32	I Should Have Known Better	Casual #9 — Long Ride
05:16	Can't Buy Me Love	Casual #14 — The Stake
07:28	And I Love Her	Casual #5 — Silk Crossover
09:58	Help!	Casual #19 — Pelvic Punch
12:17	You've Got to Hide Your Love Away	Casual #20 — Pelvic Wave
14:26	Ticket to Ride	Casual #26 — The Hurdler
17:32	Magical Mystery Tour	Casual #34 — Sweep Wing
20:20	Start Me Up	Intimate #2 — I See the Light
23:45	Hang Fire	Intimate #3 — The Hip Twist
26:07	Slave	Intimate #8 — Knee Claps
31:05	Little T & A	Intimate #16 — Side Splitters
34:31	Black Limousine	Intimate #23 — Pelvic Pushups
38:06	Neighbors	Intense #4 — Frogleg Backstroke
41:42	Heartbreaker	Intense #10 — Heel Play
45:58	(She's Just a Woman)	Intense #7 — Split Sideways
48:41	Ramble On	Intense #14 — Ceiling Touch
53:23	Moby Dick	Intimate #35 — Leg Snaps
57:46	Bring It on Home	Casual #8 — Tongue Lashes
62:03	The End	Take a deep breath and walk it off

LABORS OF LOVE

This series times out to 38:30 for working out to one of the most popular record albums of all time: *Saturday Night Fever*. The concentration here is on the Intimate Level Sexercises, and the sequence starts easy and works up to two Intense Sexercises, and then comes back down, like a bell-shaped curve. With this one, try to get into the music and the beat. Turn the music up and soak it up as you get into yourself and feel parts of your body responding to both the music and the exercising.

Artist: The Bee Gees & Others
Album: Saturday Night Fever
Record Company: RSO Records
Album's Serial Number: RS-2-4001
Side: One and Three

The Sexercises

Timer	Song	Sexercise
00:01	Stayin' Alive	Casual #5 — Silk Crossover
04:47	How Deep Is Your Love?	Intimate #2 — Tunnel of Love
08:54	Night Fever	Intimate #3 — Hip Twist
12:28	More Than a Woman	Intimate #11 — The Delicate Butterfly
15:46	If I Can't Have You	Intense #8 — Split Sideways Supreme
18:45	Night on Disco Mountain	Intense #3 — The Bloom
23:57	Open Sesame	Intimate #12 — The Petals
28:00	Jive Talkin'	Intimate #21 — The Pelvic Thrust I
32:01	You Should Be Dancin'	Intimate #19 — The Wedge Leg
36:15	Boogie Shoes	Casual #39 — Hippie-Hippie Shake
38:30	The End	

WHITE FIRE

There have been many singers who have built their careers on doing love songs — songs that stir emotion, that create images, that lull the listener into moods of passion and love. Johnny Mathis has been one of the most consistent performers in the business in creating a mood of love. White Fire lasts only fifteen minutes and forty-eight seconds, and it is all Casual Level Sexercises, but for a lights-turned-down kind of workout on a night filled with warmth, it is excellent. It is also excellent for an intimate night at home, with the lights down and the music up. Make your lover comfortable, put this side on and go through the five Sexercises slowly and deliberately, losing a little more clothing after each one. You lover can wait until the fifteen minutes are over — can't he?

Artist: Johnny Mathis
Album: The First 25 Years
Record Company: Columbia
Album's Serial Number: C2X-37440
Side: Three

The Sexercises

Timer	Song	Sexercise
00:01	Chances Are	Casual #9 — The Long Ride
03:04	All the Things You Are	Casual #4 — Feline Stretch
06:41	A Time for Us	Casual #38 — The Sway
09:38	Nothing Between Us But Love	Casual #17 — Sphinx Drop
13:02	There! I've Said It Again	Casual #3 — Double Tuck
15:48	The End	

SEXERCISE AND YOU

From the time we conceived the book you've just read, we had it in mind as a book where the reader very much takes part in its ideas and concepts. Sort of a two-way book, between the two of us. I'd like to take the entire process one step farther by asking you to fill in the following questionnaire so that I can get your feedback on how the book worked or did not work for you. I know that I hate to damage a book, so if you'd rather not tear this one apart but still want to fill in the questionnaire for me, Xerox this page and send it to me. We plan on using the information for an article in an upcoming issue of *Fit* magazine. If you'd like to check out a copy of *Fit* in the meantime, send one dollar to *Fit,* P.O. Box 493, Murray Hill Station, New York, NY 10157, and mention that I promised you a sample copy if you'd cover postage and handling. Looking forward to hearing from you.

— Kym Herrin

About You

Sex: ☐ Male ☐ Female

Age: ☐ Below 21 ☐ 21-29 ☐ 30-39 ☐ 40-49 ☐ 50-59 ☐ 60 or over

Fitness: ☐ Very fit ☐ Fit ☐ Getting fit ☐ Need work

Marital status: ☐ Single ☐ Divorced ☐ Widowed ☐ Living with someone

Do you consider yourself: ☐ Liberal-minded ☐ Middle-of-the-road ☐ Conservative
☐ Very conservative

Did you enjoy the book? ☐ Yes ☐ No

Who bought the book? ☐ I purchased it ☐ A friend bought it for me

Do you agree with the book's philosophy? ☐ Yes ☐ No

Have you made use of the book at this point? ☐ Yes ☐ No

Have you begun a regular Sexercise program? ☐ Yes ☐ Now

If Sexercise classes were offered in your area, would you attend? ☐ Yes ☐ No

Would you be interested in another Sexercise book? ☐ Yes ☐ No

If you answered Yes to the previous question, would you like the next book to be in one of the following formats? ☐ A workbook of exercises and positions ☐ More plain talk about how to put the Sexercises to use ☐ A Sexercise book on developing beauty and poise ☐ A book of advice and information for active women in a question-and-answer format ☐ A book that would take the Sexercist concept a next big step

☐ Other: _____

We'd like you to share with us what you felt about this book. Did it help you? Did it serve to make your sex more frequent or of better quality? Did it help improve your self-esteem? Did it inspire you to a fitness program you'd been contemplating? Give us your reaction to what the book did for you in your own words:

_____

_____

_____

_____

Name: _____ Phone: _____

Address: _____ City _____

State: _____ ZIP: _____

☐ You may use my name in the article ☐ Please do not use my name

(Return the questionnaire to: The Sexercise Book, Anderson World Inc., 1400 Stierlin Road, Mountain View, CA 94043.)